BAREFOOT SOUL
Runner's Handbook

The Brain Sole Connection

CSABA LUCAS

"Csaba Lucas shares a comprehensive revisit to our natural, primal nature and the health and freedom available to us all through a natural approach to running and connecting with Mother Earth.

This is NOT a book full of "tech-talk" and statistics from biomechanical studies of robots and stick figures as so many are, but is a book of Truth-Talk on the facts of life, running, and how to be healthy and stay connected to the reality of life on earth."

– Paul Chek, Founder of the Chek Institute and a world-renowned expert in the fields of corrective and high-performance exercise kinesiology

"In this valuable handbook for barefoot running Csaba Lucas has captured the essence of the relationship of human movement and the human soul. His passion speaks clearly in every page of this informative and inspiring handbook for runners of all ages and abilities. Beyond the why and how humans propel themselves over this earth, Csaba has communicated the freedom of spirit that comes with barefoot running with a blend of science and the understandings of a master technician.

This book will make any runner healthier."

– Robert Forster, Sports Medicine Physical Therapist to 60 Olympic medalists including sprinters Allyson Felix and Jackie Joyner

"You know it's always a good time to reconnect to the primal you, the you before the shoe, and there is no quicker way to restart this connection than by taking off your shoes and reexperiencing the default you, the one your parents gave you, the one before you've added anything. Let the Barefoot Soul Running Handbook be a guiding tool you use to take yourself to the next level of you that has been waiting to be rediscovered and reactivated. If my life has anything to demonstrate, it's that the simplest things nourish us deeply.

You and your bare feet standing on the ground breathing fresh air with sun on your face is a first good step for a life of health and well-being. Start today. The adventure lasts a lifetime."

**– Barefoot Ted, legendary ultra-distance runner
from the bestselling book *'Born to Run'***

"Though I love colorful running shoes, after reading 'Barefoot Soul', I might part with them once in a while."

**– László Kalmár Nagy, National record holder of
multiple ultra-distance running races in Hungary**

connect with me
@coachbarefoot.com

To my wife, Winter

"...just us and the wild..."

CONTENTS

9   Foreword

13   1. A Running Relationship

19   2. The Story of Persistence Running

25   3. The Tool of Persistence Running

27   4. Barefoot Skin

33   5. Barefoot Restricted

35   6. Mixed Footwear

38   7. Consider Clothing

42   8. Additional Surprising Benefits

45   9. Competition and Other Pitfalls

49   10. For competitive Athletes

      11. Breathing and Speed

55   12. Foot Landing

61   13. The Unity of the Body Parts

71   14. Stretching & Massaging

72   15. Extra Conditioning Exercises

76   16. Hazards & Signs

78   17. Duality in Recovery

81   18. Relationship between Walking,
          Running and Doing

84   19. Child Passions, Relationships &
          Communal Running

88   20. In Closing

91   I Progressive barefoot development

96   II Runner's basic supporting exercises

105   III Runner's basic stretches

121   IV Acknowledgements

123   Disclaimer

125   About the Author

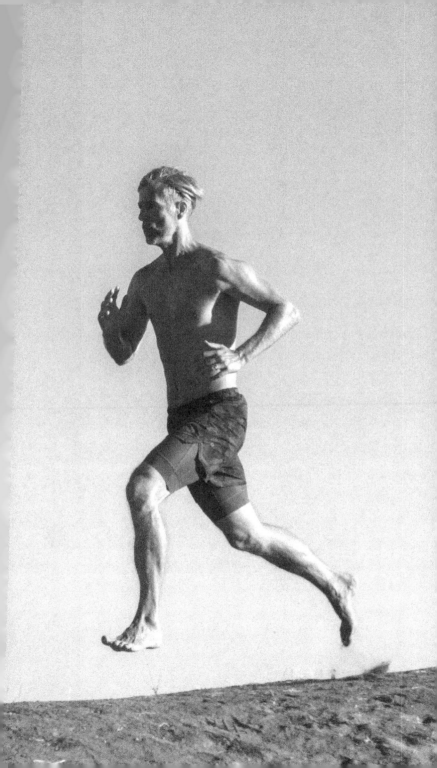

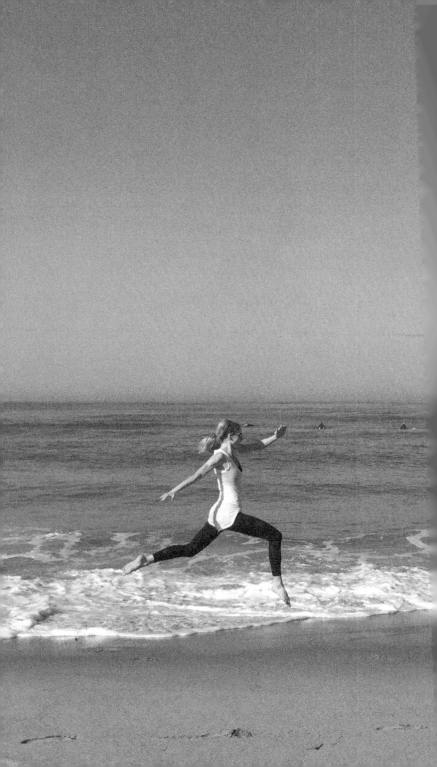

FOREWORD

Running has been an integral part of my life since my teens. Somehow, for some reason, I felt running was calling to me, pulling me in, promising me something I knew I needed, but wasn't even myself sure what exactly, or why. I finally put a pair of running shoes on, walked down the driveway, looked down the long, country road I grew up on, enticing me to see what was waiting for me once I would take those first few strides. Slowly gaining speed, legs pumping, lungs expanding, I realized what I had been longing for: clarity.

Running quickly became a passion, almost an obsession (if not fully an obsession). I was addicted. I was running every day, flying down the long tree lined roads, through rain or shine, snow and high heat; nothing deterred me. I needed to run like I needed the air I was breathing. It became my solace in life. I was at peace, I was grounded, I was present and thoughtful. Running became my therapy.

I continued on my running path ever since, always making it a priority; I was never too busy to fit a run in, whatever was going on. I even ran throughout both of my pregnancies, safely and doctor-approved, my ever-growing belly only making me more determined to carry on.

In my early twenties as life became more complicated, I joined a gym for convenience and hit the treadmills. When I didn't have time to get out into the hills of Los Angeles, it was a quick way to get my "fix". I could feel it wasn't the same as being outside in nature, but when I had no choice, I was totally fine to settle. Eventually, I began having a shooting pain in my knee, specifically when I was using the treadmill. In the beginning, I powered through it, certain it would go away as quickly as it came on. Of course, it didn't. I started running with a knee compression brace, which helped a little bit, but I couldn't help thinking "this can't be right". I was suddenly faced with the fate I knew many runners have had to deal with at some point in their running careers; I had to stop running or face up to the possibility of knee surgery. I feared that it was the only way out and back to running. But, instead, I took a pause and listened to my most basic wisdom and I stepped off the treadmill, indefinitely, and committed myself exclusively to the dusty, rocky hills I loved running so much. Though the knee pain disappeared, I had some on and off ankle problems, which I decided to learn to live with.

When I met my husband, Csaba, the author of this book, and the coach-of-all-things-health-related, he had a difficult task in front of him: changing the way I looked at and approached running. I listened to what he had to say, but it was hard for me to wrap my mind around his philosophies. He felt there was something bigger to running, something even more basic, simpler, that me and most runners were confused by in our information and consumerism filled world. His findings were backed by his many decades of practical experience, and his successful mentoring guidance towards other runners of all levels. The center piece of his message was barefoot running. I couldn't accept the idea of running barefoot. It seemed scary and painful, and I saw it as a hindrance to my already well-oiled routine. I had my way, and he did his own things differently, as he always does. However, I started to question myself: was I the one who was doing things differently and maybe he was the one doing things the way we are all meant to do? We were equally passionate about health and running, but he and his mentees had no pains and frustrations attached to their favorite physical activities.

Under his wing, he got me to reactivate my body in a way that was (there is no other way to say it) more natural. Since I was too scared to be a full-time barefoot runner, Csaba gradually introduced me to the FiveFinger minimalist running shoes. I'll never forget the first time I wore them out and got some 'proper participation' from my feet into my movement. We went for a hike together and I can still remember the feeling. It felt liberating! It was like a massage on my feet. I loved the feeling and I was hooked. I was satisfied with my mostly FiveFinger shoe experience, but Csaba was only more motivated in continuing the push towards simplicity.

I personally had a hard time diving all the way into barefoot running, but I go on barefoot hikes, and I've incorporated many of the wisdoms in this book into a part of my running and health procedures. One thing I learned from my experiences and from being around Csaba and from being barefoot, was that I could incorporate certain aspects and still reap the benefits. The system is not about being 'all or nothing'; one doesn't need to be a purist to significantly improve overall well-being. This running handbook is something that every runner, no matter if they're barefoot or in shoes, can refer to for information and inspiration. The content is timeless, and can be passed down for generations to come, equally beneficial today as it will be in the future. It's an ancient way of being that is still applicable to our modern-day wired bodies. You don't have to have an all or nothing approach! Implementing these ideas gradually will also be beneficial. Csaba's message provides the clarity many runners are looking for, and provides some basic wisdom about running, which is still mostly unknown in our modern world.

You may start out only wanting to walk barefoot, and that's fine! One day you might change your mind and decide you're ready for more! As someone who is very passionate about running, I can safely say you will find inspiration in this handbook that will resonate with you in one way, and as you get better, or more adventurous, the book will eventually resonate with you in a different way. It is a book to keep referring to.

What I realized about this handbook is that, barefoot or not, running is a passion for so many people and this book was written for those who love running. It's more than a book about running barefoot. It truly is an informational guide for the discovery and maintenance of the runners' body and psyche. Whether you desire to run barefoot, or already are a barefoot runner, whether you're a professional runner or new to the game; this book simply speaks to the runner's soul.

WINTER AVE ZOLI

(a mother, running partner, wife, best friend, writer and some other things)
August 5, 2021 Los Angeles

BAREFOOT SOUL

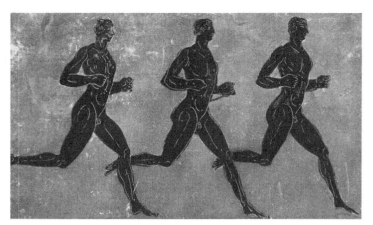

Runners on ancient Greek ceramic vessels, circa 330 BC

1. A RUNNING RELATIONSHIP

People love to run. Humans developed a love for running way before pre-written history, and we can witness the fascination with running through art and artifacts dating all the way back to ancient Greek times, with a modern resurrection in the 1980's, and probably with the most popularity, today. Jogging and trail running are the most consistently popular outdoor sports practiced in the United States, and one of the fastest growing sports in the modern world.

Running on a regular schedule is what a vast majority of people associate with being in shape, or at least that it is a means for getting into better shape. There is substantial research on the subject of running that points to its significant role in our evolutionary development. Our upright posture, sweat glands, Achilles-tendons, feet, neck and dozens of other body parts evolved to enable us to run long, even ultra-long distances making humans the best 'distance runner' mammals of the animal kingdom.

Yet, according to most statistics, approximately 80% of the people who run regularly suffer from some type of running related injuries. These statistics do not even address the psychological burn out that can occur in recreational 'ex-runners', or even in many professional athletes.

In my 38 years of running and nearly three decades of coaching, I've come full circle with running. I went from being a champion runner to someone who hated running. I despised, even warned against the pitfalls of the sport. Eventually, after doing a lot of research, I learned about the importance of running from ancient hunter gatherer societies, and finally discovered how to run in a way that actually helped people to physically heal, get into better shape and through the practicing of running, even develop a better balance between social and work life.

This handbook was not written in a lab, nor is it based on 'black and white' information. I decided to use an approach, which I would like to see as a reader in books: personal, viscerally tested approaches put into practice by a large variety of people all over the world from many different cultures, with some current scientific facts tacked on, when suitable. In this book you will see some references to research and studies, but I am not a big fan of sticking to scientific information. Science represents only the current understanding of a subject, which in terms of running doesn't yield to much inspiration, fun, nor sustainable processes. I put a reference guide of books and resources at the end of this handbook, which can lead you in many different directions, in the case you are interested in further investigating the scientific aspect of the subject of barefoot running.

When I was 8 years old, I began running as part of a standard regiment that every Eastern European athlete went through, regardless of one's main sport. Back in the 1980's my first and now highly-accomplished canoeing coach, Robert Weiss, always said 'running is the base of all sports'. Robert and the world of athletics, directed by sophisticated sports science, much of which originated from the Soviet athlete development system, were correct. I developed pretty decent capabilities, without ever focusing on running. As a youngster, I became one of the top three in my school's sprinting championship, then at age 15, I won the 800-meter county running championship, and on the side, I regularly ran half-Marathons as part of my extra-curricular training for canoeing. I did not end up venturing down the Olympic path in canoeing - unlike many of my champion teammates. I loved the multi-sport aspect of canoe training, the weekly swimming, weightlifting, gymnastics, soccer, handball, and of course the canoeing, but I couldn't stand the running. Even though I was a good runner, I grew to hate running as a teenager. The commonly used running principles expected athletes to keep improving their running performance at a rate that I, personally, was not able to sustain, psychologically. Once I quit canoeing, I was happy to swear that I would never run again in my life. I turned my attention to other sports and became a county champion in discus tossing, shot-put, and regional champion in obstacle course biking, multiple wins in city obstacle course championships, and I won some random dancing competitions. Once I got into weightlifting seriously, I even became an Airplane Pull Champion in Courtenay, Canada; the goal being to see who could pull a military airplane the fastest for 100 yards. I competed in kickboxing briefly, studied ballet, rock climbed, practiced yoga and tai chi regularly and learned fencing. I experimented with the human body's capabilities. I also studied the science of Olympic weightlifting, kinesthesiology, massage therapy, and interned for years in chiropractic care, physiotherapy and acupuncture. I was curious to discover how to create the best and healthiest body one could have, in order to enjoy a long and vital life.

In the early 90's, along the way in my journey through sports, I was educated by some highly renowned health gurus in North America. The ideas they preached in regards to long distance running perfectly fit my experience. The bottom line always boiled down to a few seemingly solid points. Since even the fastest humans couldn't run away from a dangerous animal, it seemed from an evolutionary stand point pretty obvious to conclude that there were no upsides to focusing on improvement in running capabilities. The sceptics also pointed out that strong, muscular bodies developed from weightlifting not from long distancing running, which gives rise to wiry, skinny bodies. The argument was simple, which one of those bodies seemed more attractive? Also, based on legitimate running related injury statistics, running seemed to have major negative effects on people, which I easily related to, and for our musculo-skeletal system it seemed just straight-up bad for people to run. I also eagerly agreed with this information because I was psychologically scarred by running, and up to that point, could only see the downside. It didn't help either that in the 80's and 90's era of muscular pop culture heroes were the likes of Arnold Schwarzenegger, Sylvester Stallone, Bruce Willis and many others who seemed like anything but runners.

I succeeded in coaching and created a company that delivered the expected results to both champion athletes and to the sedentary individuals wanting to get into better shape.

My outlook on running was tested when I met my wife, who is an avid runner. I managed not to get infected by her love of running for a while, but I was envious of the joy she carried in anticipation of her runs out in nature. Eventually, I decided to try running again. The popular running spot in my neighborhood in Brooklyn was a track around a park. I ran around the park the way I knew how to run; all guns blazing. I managed to pass every single runner, but by the end of the run I was back at the same place as before: I hated running. But I could not get running out of my mind. There had to be something to it, if someone who I valued as much as my wife loved this activity, not to mention all the other passionate and smart runners I knew. I decided to dissect running scientifically to a point where I could first make sense of it for myself in my mind, and then eventually perhaps incorporate practicing it differently than I ever had. Since I had a small research group available at my company, gathering a variety of substantial information was easy. I went at it to find out what I was doing wrong, what was I missing? Surprisingly, I got to the core of my issues fast. As an athlete I learned to run in the same way that the modern 'ever growing' world approached everything; 'Bigger, better, faster'. This realization freed my mind up immediately, because that was

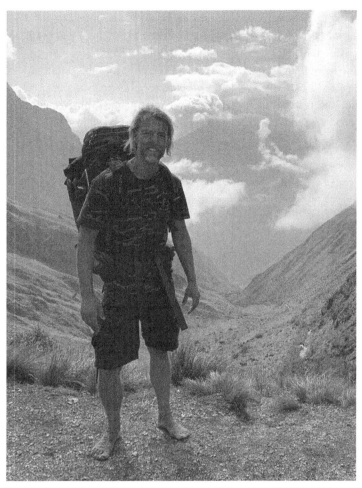

Coaching in my preferred office, nature... wearing only FYF socks, at 18,000 feet in the Peruvian Andes

obviously an unrealistic goal as a human being. My curiosity about running grew substantially and I quickly realized that it was not only I who was getting injured psychologically, many runners physically as well. Most of the running world, as I discovered, is to some degree, 'injured'.

At the same time, all of the research led me to the conclusion that we, as a human species, were designed to run. So, I was again confused, but this was a good type of confusion. I knew that I was onto something. I decided to look at running from the simplest view and I had two realizations: Firstly, sprinters train as if they are cheetahs, but they are not. Secondly, long distance runners train like racehorses, and just like racehorses, they are getting injured.

It dawned on me that people are in the need to run the way human beings were designed to run, and not how the modern world dictates us to run - faster, quicker and better. We are meant to run the way our persistence hunting ancestors ran.

Persistence hunting was a very successful hunting method during which humans used their superior endurance capabilities to run down kudus, elands and other large antelopes in Africa until the prey collapsed in sheer physical exhaustion. Through the process of persistence hunting, a necessary skill of the hunter was to be a great tracker, but what allowed the tracking skill to yield to success was the way the hunter persistently ran after the animal. This, indeed, was the human style of running, Persistence Running!

In this handbook I will outline what principles one needs to keep in mind to learn, develop, sustain and master Persistence Running, in a way that will aid the runner for the rest of their lives without breaking down their bodies in the process. This way of running has multiple positive side effects in my experience, some scientifically proven, and many, which science has yet to prove. I have seen those unproven, uplifting side effects over and over during the past few decades. Science seems to be always one step behind in understanding the processes that master practitioners know, without scientific proof. The fun, yet-to-be proven side effects of barefoot Persistence Running are: anti-aging, happiness, a renewed connection to nature, enlarged brain capacity, and a deeper sense of grounding via 'earthing'.

My goal with this book is to motivate you, the reader (regardless of your current skill level as a runner), to start to practice Persistence Running. If you stay persistent with your practices (no pun intended), then these efforts will lead you to discover how to use your body's capabilities, and gradually evolve to learn to pass that unpredictable point in running, which most people refer to as 'hitting a wall'. You might even organically build up to the 'ultradistances' all humans evolved to be able to cover. On your path of practice, you will learn how it truly feels to be a human being. It is not about the speed, nor the pace, nor really about the distance. It is all about a human experience spiced with enlightening realizations along the way, building the foundation for a lifetime of running.

2. THE STORY OF PERSISTENCE RUNNING

In your mind, go back 15,000 years. Imagine the following: A tribe is hunting. One tribesman "sprints" after the prey. The prey escapes, but the sprinter and the tribe follow – the escape is temporary. The main runner and the tribe always stay close enough that the prey can never fully recover from its sprint. The tribe keep at it. When the group gets close enough to the prey, the main runner sprints at it again, scaring the prey out of the shade during the high heat of the savannah. They repeat this process persistently, over and over, until eventually the prey collapses from exhaustion. The animal is then killed with a rock, or a spear.

The theory that persistence hunting played a crucial part in the evolution of man was first suggested only in 1984 by David Carrier. We were unaware of this type of hunting in the western world for a very long time. Though our ancestors practiced this type of hunting, the skill and the stories were not passed down to our modern civilization, and was lost somewhere along the twists and turns of western history. The main concept was based on the observation that man is one of the only mammals that cools off by sweating. Most four-legged mammals pant to cool themselves, but they are physically unable to pant while they run.

In conclusion, if our early human ancestors could chase an animal long enough, the animal would eventually overheat, collapsing in heat exhaustion. Humans were then able to kill it with relative ease.

This theory was advanced by the Harvard paleoanthropologist Daniel Lieberman. Lieberman wrote a substantial amount on the subject explaining that based on anatomical, genetic, and paleontological evidence, there are an overwhelming number of features in the human body that make us good at running. Furthermore, many of these physiological characteristics have no other function, but clearly indicate humans were selected for long distance running. He has noted that those features — for example the arched feet, short toes, wide shoulders, long Achilles' tendons — seem to have originated around two million years ago, right around the time when our ancestors began accessing meat as a regular part of a new style of hominin diet. Persistence hunting, he's argued, might have been the evolutionary driver.

These ideas came to the attention of the now popular author Christopher McDougall, who brought up and somewhat

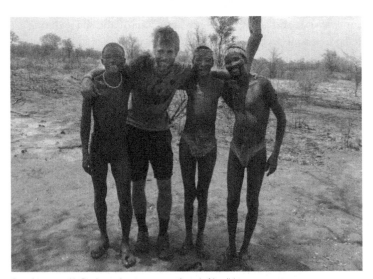

On a journey with Bushman hunters somewhere in Namibia

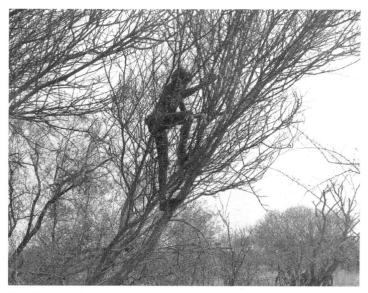

Elder Bushman collecting sap

popularized the theory in his book about endurance running, "Born to Run," which became a bestseller in 2009. McDougall backed up the theory with concrete evidence about the Mexican Tarahumara tribe, in regards to the theoretical human capabilities identified by Lieberman. McDougall concluded that this explains why we like to run marathons, even ultra-marathons, and are fairly good at it. When we run distances, he implied, we are fulfilling our biological destiny.

During the past four decades I have had the good fortune to witness and experience these running related theoretical ideas in real life. Besides running a substantial amount, I also spent an extended amount of time living and hunting amongst hunter-gatherers in Africa and South America. My exposure and experiences, particularly with the San tribe of Botswana and Namibia, gave me a front row seat to learning and practicing with some of the last persistence hunters. In my experience, the way the San spend their lives is truly extraordinary from a physical standpoint. One of the big surprises for me was how much they actually move.

The tribe wakes up with the sun at around 5:30 am, and pull a fire together; they smoke some tobacco, clean their weapons, and by 7:00 am they are on their way to hunt and gather. Their movement is always at least a well-paced walk. This means that it is not a leisurely paced activity but rather movement with a purpose. They have all of their weapons and a survival kit with them at all times: one spear, a bow with about 10 poisonous arrows, two wood sticks designated

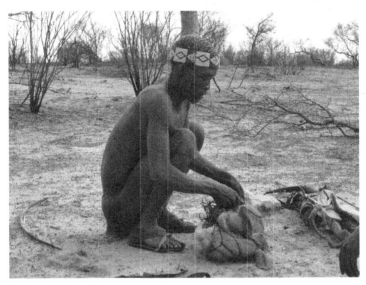

Bushman Hunter packing up prey

to light a fire, some sort of tobacco, a digging stick, and some tiny, multi-purpose rope. Since they don't take water or food with them, whenever they see an opportunity, they snack (for example on a particular tree sap, which requires some tree-handling, since it is up high, and awkward to get to). If they come across it, they also dig out edible roots, some of these are like giant potatoes filled with watery fibers. These roots are often hidden 3 feet deep, and it can easily take 20 minutes of intensive digging to get to the edible parts.

Generally, during the hunt, the San keep themselves focused so if an opportunity arises and a prey animal comes into sight, they can actively pursue it (but only if the wind is blowing from the direction of the animal). They might see some animal tracks, which make sense to follow. At this point they will split their attention between following the tracks, which I could barely see, let alone follow, and looking around constantly for the presence of other potential prey.

Humans have developed many different hunting styles and the San utilizes all of them, given the season and the circumstances. Sometimes when there is prey nearby, everyone becomes more still than even the most highly trained hunting dog. One of the hunters goes down onto hands and knees and crawls as close to the prey as possible, attempting to take down the animal with a poisonous arrow. If they succeed, they wrap up the whole animal and carry it home on their backs.

At other times of the year, when the new rain has softened up the ground after the dry season, they might decide to run down animals, and practice persistence hunting. During the main part of the persistence hunt, the persistence running is well paced and induced with sprints to scare the animal as they close in on it. The persistence hunt can last anywhere from about two to nine hours long.

The San also look at traps, which they set out days before. Building a trap requires collecting some wood sticks and branches, setting the pieces up like an intricate puzzle, and making some rope out of plant fibers (which is also a physical activity requiring concentrated focus).

Mid-day when the temperature is very high, they rest for about one hour, cleaning, sharpening their weapons, day dreaming or napping. They then continue with their pursuit, running and walking until the sun starts to set.

When they arrive back to the camp at the end of the day, they gather on the dirt ground and eat a large meal together.

Traditionally in the evening, they light a big campfire, and based on what they managed to gather or hunt, the women sing and the men dance around in a semi-trance. The dancing is all done with the lower part of the body only, no arm gestures. Their feet seemingly move so little, but the movement is so skilled and fast, that though I consider myself a good dancer and athlete, I never managed to figure out how to follow them. At the absolute latest, the tribe is off to sleep around 9:00 pm.

The next day everything starts all over again. This goes on every day, during a non-existent week, all along a non-existent year. You might think that this is monotonous, but nothing is further from the truth. The San are amongst their loved ones, together with their best friends all day long, in an ever-changing natural environment that they know intricately and love intimately.

The point of my description is to give you an understanding of how active we human beings are meant to be. With this lifestyle it is no surprise that all of the hunter-gatherers possess the capability to run extreme distances.

Unfortunately, this past decade did not favor the left-over persistence hunters. Based on my conversations with my San persistence hunting teachers, their sons and daughters have not been interested in learning all the intricate knowledge required to learn persistence hunting. The new generation would rather pursue hunting that requires less physical activity (for example, clubbing porcupine). This way, they can turn some of their attentions towards connecting to the modern, outside world by trying to acquaint themselves with devices (mostly cell phones) as a newly found channel to a world the San of previous generations decided not to embrace. According to the book "Affluence Without Abundance", written by James Suzman, the San stopped hunting as persistence hunters during this past decade. Based on my experience, I still believe that even today a few deeply hidden tribes practice this beautiful running spectacle of human capability.

Part of my motivation in writing this book is to put my learnings out to the modern world and inspire you, the reader, to connect to a modern version of persistence hunting, and start practicing Persistence Running. This ancient human skill can be kept alive by us, at least in part.

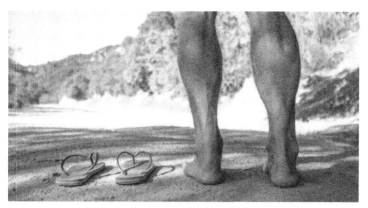

Leaving the flip flops behind

3. THE TOOL OF
PERSISTENCE RUNNING

During a Persistence Run, you run with your entire body, brain included. You need to use everything available to you from within yourself, if you intend to keep a healthy running career that will last a lifetime.

Have you ever observed when a dog is taken off the leash, how it speeds around in circles, full of joy? That is the sense of freedom and joy people need to aim towards discovering in physical activities, especially in running.

Presently, the single most restrictive item people put on for movement are shoes. Shoes are limiting many aspects of movement, contrary to common belief. The many small bridges in the foot, the joints, the muscles and the skin cannot do their intended jobs when covered and restricted. Furthermore, the limited capability of the foot makes the entire body move drastically different by overcompensating and altering its natural design. Your feet and your body are the technology. It's not the shoe, nor any of the other equipment, as most large shoe and outfitting manufacturing companies would like us to believe.

I will cut to the chase: there is no way to run, walk or even move properly, not only as a Persistence Runner, but also as a human being, as long as you wear shoes. Until the day babies are born with shoes on their feet this will remain to be the case.

Of course, people in our modern world wear shoes, love shoes and are not about to give up shoes any time soon. I personally enjoy shoes as well. Perhaps finding a middle ground, a balance between a "shoe-less" and "shoe-full" life could bring much benefit to all of us.

There are some activities that neither you, nor me, would ever want to do without shoes. But there are plenty of other things we should NOT do in shoes, if we want to have the best performance, while feeling our best and getting injured less.

I am aware that there are different types of people who are interested in barefoot existence for different reasons. This handbook will outline how and what you can do to bring in the right practice of barefoot activities into your life, and feel 'comfortable' during the process. Overtime your ideas might change in regards to being barefoot, but for now, let's try to find your entry point into the barefoot world.

Being barefoot at home is nice, but it is a far cry from doing anything substantial for your body, or your mind. You might have the desire to learn running barefoot, but that might be too big of a step from where you are right now. You may find that walking barefoot is the proper first step for you, or exercising barefoot, but you also might be someone who is capable to start experimenting immediately with running barefoot. I encourage you to be patient and persistent with your new practices rather than fast, which can often lead to discouragement (and possibly injury). Set out for the process to last a lifetime, instead of focusing simply on getting on track, or trying to perform better for next month's race.

So, let's dive into this, bare feet first! We will learn what all the information means in practical terms, and eventually how to apply it to exercises, exercise programs and running!

4. BAREFOOT SKIN

The soles of your feet are covered with a very special type of skin. This miraculous skin is highly pressure sensitive, even when it is callused up. According to related research, there is no difference in the foots' sole skin sensitivity, whether people's feet are thick with callouses, or if the pedicurist keeps them smooth and soft.

Nature's shoes – the highly pressure sensitive skin on your foot- has a high amount of proprioceptors, which send information to your brain about the surface with which your feet are connecting. The proprioceptors of your feet are meant to be your eyes on the ground.

The brain is a key player in most things we do, and operating our body while running barefoot is no different. Every part of the brain works under the motto 'use it or lose it'. When your brain does not receive sufficient information from your feet about the ground's surface, your brain slowly shuts down on this function, as there is no need for it to be alert. When the part of the brain that evolved to translate the large variety of surfaces our bodies might operate upon is not used, that part of the brain goes into hibernation. This

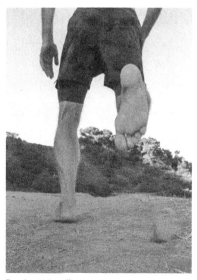

process is similar to the synaptic pruning your brain experiences when using a GPS instead of a more traditional map - leading to an overall decreased spatial cognitive capability. The part of the brain that is in 'hibernation' will affect many related functions. In terms of the feet constantly being enclosed in shoes, the related functions are the movement of the entire body.

Barefoot take-off

Luckily, the brain has neuroplasticity, which is the ability of neural networks in the brain to change through growth and reorganization at any age.

In our practical experience the more barefoot movement is used the more versatile messages the proprioceptors are sending to the brain, resulting in elevated sensory communication and use of the brain. The "barefoot" brain is forced to stay awake and send ever changing instructions to the body in regards to gait length (length of step), type of foot landing, arm and shoulder movement, and even spinal curvature and rotation, with many more overwhelming combinations of ways the body can move.

Running on a trail with sharp pebbles requires a drastically different style of running than running on grass, or running on sand, rocks, or asphalt. Not only is it the geographical surface that affects the way the body moves, but every individual step is different without shoes on a natural surface – the body's weight distribution changes according to what is below the foot - one, or five, or ten pebbles.

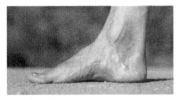
Barefoot athlete's foot

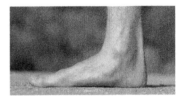
Shoed athlete's foot

When you step on a rock your brain 'knows' about the rock because the proprioceptors sense that particular rock and the instructions it sends to the body, causing you to shift your weight away from your normal center of gravity, while still keeping stability. This reaction, for instance, helps you to avoid twisted ankles (which can be very common in thick soled shoes for trail running). This is the reason you will hardly, if ever, twist your ankle while being barefoot. My wife had severe ankle sprains until she switched to alternative, minimalist shoed and shoeless running regiments. This is the same reason why experienced, solely barefoot runners feel unstable while running in shoes. Have you ever witnessed what happens to a cat or dog when someone puts shoes on their feet? It is somewhat of a disturbing sight, because the animal cannot sense the ground below its feet either, resulting in awkward body movements. Of course, dogs and cats can also get used to it, but that doesn't mean they won't suffer from similar issues as shoe wearing humans.

One day, while I was horseback riding, my expert riding partner told me that when they train mustangs and later ride them in the mountains, the mustangs can go down steep, rocky hills without any issues, but stable raised horses always need to look at their feet to be able to manage the difficult surface. Horses with horseshoes have no sense of the ground either.

Beginner and intermediate barefoot runners also experience 'foot blindness'; indeed, one of the signs of a master barefoot runner is that they do not need to look down constantly while running, because they learned how to 'see' with their feet and they trust their body's capability to adjust to surface changes as they come.

In my running community's experience, the more the bare foot is used, the more the runner can feel with their feet even while not running, and even more surprisingly, the more sensitive the skin on the foot becomes. Yes, it seems counter intuitive to people who have no experience in barefoot existence, but the more you are on your bare feet, the more sensitive your foot skin will become, even as calluses and a thicker skin develop!

Once you throw your running shoes away and commit to barefoot running, you will develop some more calluses, but not nearly as much as you think you will. Your foot will transform gradually, but not in the way most people expect it to.

The skin on the sole will not change significantly, but the 'meatiness' and the thickness of the bottom of your foot will change. The muscles in your feet will also become more robust, and your arch will rise higher.

Usually, people experience a shrinking foot size as their feet get conditioned, because as the arch becomes more prominent and lifts up, the foot shortens; just as if you pinched a piece of rope from the ground – the rope shortens its foot print. Your foot size will always change based on how much you run. Later, once you have developed some serious skills in barefoot running, during extremely active running seasons your foot can actually swell up - sometimes even adding two extra sizes. During normal seasons your feet will always shrink back down to their usual size.

THE CONDUIT TO MOVEMENT

As you walk or run barefoot, your skin's proprioceptors constantly send messages to your brain and the brain appropriately responds with instructions on how to land the foot, what gait length to use and how to move the arms, rotate the spine, move the elbows and so on. When you have shoes on, the foot's skin proprioceptors always sense the inside of the shoe; therefore, the messages to the brain remain pretty much the same. The result of highly repetitive information from the feet leads to the brain instructing the body to move in the same way. A bored brain is more receptive to aging and to other breakdowns. Though there are scientists who are already making great strides in connecting the dots between cerebral palsy, stroke, muscular dystrophy and sarcopenia patients and people's changed gaits, science has not yet managed to confirm the scientific connection between the brain's atrophy and the body's movement. I predict that sooner or later science will catch up to what experienced barefoot runners already feel; the brain and the entire nervous system's health are tightly connected to the constantly changing input from the environment – at least partially from the foot's proprioceptors. After all, the only parts of the body that are directly connected to the environment are the feet (excluding the air touching the skin, of course).

An alert and active brain will stay responsive. The surrounding environment affects the human system drastically - science is aware of this already as part of the nature vs. nurture conversation. Epigenetics has already shed some light on how the environment shapes an organism by having a large variety of receptors feeding the organism with information on how to 'shape shift' to best fit its environment. The feet are certainly an important receptor, in many regards, because by sensing the ground with which we connect to our conscious environment, it guides the rest of the body on how to adjust its self to operate the most effectively. How much nurturing of the body is due to our actual connection to the ground and its effect on the connection between our inner and outer environment is still up for discovery. However, before science discovers it you can experience it via your own body being barefoot, and feel how differently you connect to your outer environment without shoes.

In simple structural terms, when you don't change the way your foot lands, nor how your body moves, you will overuse a particular landing pattern. An overused, repetitive landing pattern is the reason most runners suffer from particular running related injuries; they suffer from running related overuse syndrome. This is the same type of overuse syndrome some workers experience while doing the same job over and over. The carpenter worker, who's job is to hammer nails in from morning until evening, is not going to be able to be proud of his strong arms, because he will suffer from tendonitis as a result of his overuse syndrome. Carpal tunnel syndrome is another form of the overuse of one type of movement.

Shoe bearing runners can have overuse syndrome from a certain type of landing. Based on their body's structure and its capability to function, they might first wear down their Achilles tendons, then their knees, IT-bands, hips, lower back, neck - just to list a few potential issues.

Does that mean no one should ever walk or run, in shoes? Well, this is a complex question. One thing is for sure, any amount of barefoot activity greater than zero will benefit you.

If your goal is to be healthy and use walking or running as a big part of your physical activity, then yes, you should be barefoot as much as possible while you are doing those activities. If you are a competitive athlete you can switch to complete barefoot running and only train in shoes enough so that you are still able to safely compete in shoes - in the case you still want to race in shoes, of course. Olympic champion marathon runner Abebe Bikila opted to permanently drop shoes. Further along in this handbook I will describe ways you can mix shoe running with barefoot running, in the appropriate combination, to potentially gain value from both activities in regards to competitive racing. There is some value in mentioning here that Persistence Running barefoot activities -what we were designed to practice- excludes racing others, or racing the clock, or even racing our own selves. Not racing doesn't mean you cannot develop extraordinary capabilities. My Hungarian country man Jozsef Rokob the winner of the most grueling race on Earth (30 Ironman in 30 Days around Lake Garda, Italy) only raced one other time in his entire life prior to winning this truly challenging event. I will come back to racing later.

As you can tell by now, the reason I am a big advocate of taking shoes off is because it is good for your body and not because I want you to return to your ancestry of being a caveman. There are plenty of surprising examples in the athletes of the running world, who grew up barefooted prior to becoming champion runners. In the case you are interested in barefoot stories, take a look at, arguably, the most famous 'birthplace' of world-class long-distance runners, Ngong, Kenya, or look up famous outlier barefoot champions like (my favorite) the Czech, Emil Zatopek.

5. BAREFOOT RESTRICTED

There are other reasons to 'free the foot' besides giving the proprioceptors of the skin the ability to do their job. The foot is constructed of a superbly complex mix of bridges and structures. When there is a restrictive structure present - like the shoe- this complex system developed by nature cannot do its job, and as a result, the feet will stiffen up, or even become deformed.

Today, most people's feet have the shape of a shoe, because the structure of people's feet is molded from early childhood. Who doesn't like a cute, tiny Adidas shoe on a 2-year-old? Who doesn't like a beautiful, high-heeled shoe accentuating the legs? Or who doesn't like a cool new pair of sneakers? There is a price to pay for the cuteness, beauty and coolness factors. Deformed toes pointing in odd directions, locked knees, and abnormally arched, painful lower backs are just some of the degenerative, structural changes that take place at least partially because of wearing shoes.

How much shoe wearing your body can take depends mostly on your genetics. If you have a narrow foot you are in luck, because you will be able to fit into most shoes your size without major deformations, but if you have a wider foot, your feet and toes will be squeezed and pushed in directions they were never meant to move.

The foot evolved to give back a large proportion of the force it lands with, to the next move. When the spring-like structures in the feet are restricted because of a cast (shoes) surrounding it, the feet will not be able to function properly and will fail to bounce back the appropriate amount of landing force into the next step. This does not only mean that you will be slower, but it also means your other body parts will have to make up for the restricted foot's job. The Achilles tendon is unique for our specie (even chimpanzees don't really have them). This tendon does a great job at transferring landing force into takeoff force. But when the Achilles tendon needs to work harder than normal, because it is forced to make up for what the restricted foot can't deliver, it will eventually be overused, and could lead to Achilles' tendon related injuries.

The pronation of the foot, which is the natural movement, the way it lands while walking or running, is another way the foot uses elastic energy to return the landing force partially into the next step or stride. Most shoe companies work very hard to get rid of the foot's pronation, and instead of really helping people, they create stiff, weak feet and ankles. A weakened foot and ankle structure will be dependent on the very shoes that created the weaknesses. Insoles are also used to correct a weak foots' alignment, but will only maintain or increase the foot's incapability to function on its own.

As the book 'Born to Run' puts it "the foot likes a good beating". This statement is an important one, and there is a lot of truth to it. The foot needs to be able to hit a hard surface so it can land properly, but neither the foot, nor the body like to be beaten up, which is why the body adjusts the movement so flawlessly to the given surface. When they performed experiments at Harvard University on skilled barefoot runners', they realized that the sheer forces around the knees and hips were no different than when the individual was walking or running. When you reestablish your body's capabilities and move according to its original settings, it will work more seamlessly.

Can you still wear shoes without destroying your feet? The least you can do is to make sure the shoes you wear are at least big enough that they will not crush your feet and create restrictions, any more than you have to. Most experienced runners know to buy big enough shoes, to where you could fit your own thumb in the space between the big toe and the tip of the shoe. The same principle must apply to any shoe you decide to wear. You should have a shoe that gives at least some freedom to your feet. Find shoes that are designed to work around your foot! For instance, instead of stuffing wide feet into a narrow shoe, find a shoe that comes in a wider width!

6. MIXED FOOTWEAR

Let's say you want to adjust your running routine, and are only willing to switch some things you do into a barefoot activity. For now, you are not interested to go barefoot in all walking and running activities. One way you can make this approach work without injuring yourself is by making an adjustment to your shoe wearing routines. For running and walking, you would alternate wearing at least four different types of shoes, switching them up every time you go out walking or running. For example, you could purchase a pair of running sandals (for example: Luna sandals), a pair of thick soled shoes (for example: Brook's Beast), a minimalist shoe (for example: Vibram Five Fingers), and let's say some

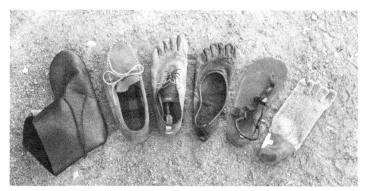

(left to right) handmade moccasin, leather sole shoe, Vibram FiveFingers (high-performance & leather), Luna Sandal, FYF sock

running sock coverings (for example: FYF Socks). Alternating footwear regularly ensures that you will not wear down any one type of landing pattern. I have seen both athletes and "weekend warriors" achieve great improvements in their physical capabilities by simply 'artificially' altering their foot's landing by using a variety of footwear. These efforts show up as a positive change to broaden the variety of ways their bodies move.

There are some warning signs you need to be aware of when switching to versatile footwear activities. When someone decides to go fully barefoot, the skin on their feet will only let them do as much as the skin on their feet can handle. The capabilities in activities performed barefoot grow gradually as the foot and skin strengthen. The skin and foot discomfort will signal when the activity is being overdone. It is relatively simple to be aware of your personal improvement in your capabilities, because you will feel comfort, as opposed to discomfort.

Once you develop a powerful and capable foot that has wired the body to move according to its proper biomechanics, you can literally wear any footwear and get away with it. Just look at the Kenyan runners who spent significant time running barefoot as youngsters and then moved on to compete in shoes. They always move as if they were running barefoot.

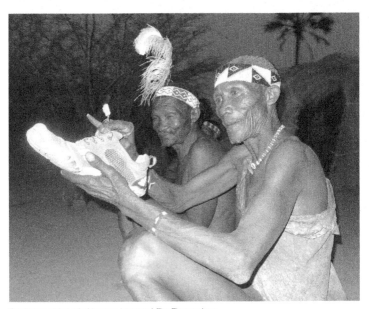

Bushman elder admiring my 'strange' FiveFinger shoe

But, in the meantime, as you begin your journey in altering a modern shoe wearing existence, and work on rewiring your system, you must be aware that some of the footwear available today could allow you to 'run yourself into the ground'.

I am personally a huge lover of the Vibram Five Finger minimalist shoes, but the combination of a thin layer of rubber between your foot and the ground, and the lack of cushioning can leave an untrained foot in a dangerous situation. If you are someone who has worn shoes all your life and have been running and walking with shoes, and in an effort to develop a more natural running style you wish to switch to wearing minimalist shoes, you need to be very cautious. The presence of the thin rubber sole will not allow the proprioceptors in your feet to regulate how hard and how much you can run with your current foot conditioning. The skin on the sole of your foot is 'protected' from the ground you are running on and you will run faster and harder than you should without the usual cushiony protection from your normal running shoes. Because minimalist shoes don't have cushioning like typical running shoes, you have to do significantly more shock absorption with your feet. It is too drastic of a change for the feet. It puts your knees, hips and lower back in jeopardy as well. Shoes like Vibram Five Fingers give your feet a false sense of protection, and if you run a longer distance than what your foot can handle without the cushioning, you are running towards some broken metatarsals; the bones in your feet. The same is true for all 'minimalist' shoes.

The problem, however, is not in the shoes, but in the imbalance amongst the capabilities of the foot, the ankles, knees, hips and lower back of the individual. Unfortunately for Vibram, the company learned about this potential danger from the many lawsuits, which were filed against them. Runners who were not educated on how to safely switch to using Vibram Five Fingers, were injuring themselves. For a healthy and strong foot conditioned to be barefoot, Vibram Five Finger footwear can be a fantastic aid in conditioning than normal running foot wear.

Until a de-conditioned foot has been properly and safely well-conditioned for barefoot/minimalist shoes, it will be better off protected by the cushion of the usual running shoe.

Here is the bottom line:

1. Going barefoot is the easiest way to balance out your body and eventually improve your capabilities, once your body (feet, ankles, etc.) has been properly conditioned.

2. If you can't fathom the idea to go completely barefoot for now, make sure to use a variety of different shoes, besides your barefoot activities.

3. Using a variety of different footwear will be a good addition to your life, even if you don't go barefoot at all.

7. CONSIDER CLOTHING

Now we know that for Persistence Running the ideal is to wear no footwear and to be barefoot.

You can also do an alternative, modern version of Persistence Running and use a big variety of foot wear on your quest towards better health and better body mechanics.

There are some other aspects of walking and running activities you need to consider. When you run barefoot, the foot stays relatively cool under normal circumstances, because the sweat glands in your feet are not covered by socks and shoes. In shoes the feet warm up and sweat disproportionately. This is the reason -according to related studies- why people who wear shoes have a much higher level of bacteria related foot skin diseases.

The number one concern people have the first time they are exposed to the idea of taking their shoes off, that I've come across, is the susceptibility to skin infections. Barefoot runners take care of their feet more than the average, due to the foot's exposure to visible dust, mud and other natural soil related substances.

Barefoot runners usually care for their feet in much more detail and use heavy-duty brushes to make sure their feet are clean. The combination of the lack of sweating inside shoes and the deep-cleaning of the feet, naturally leads to statistically significantly lower rates of infections of the skin on the feet of barefoot runners and walkers.

WARM DAYS

Most of the time when people run, the ground is cooler than their body's temperature. Running with foot skin exposed on warmer days can transfer the coolness from the ground through the body, acting as a cooling mechanism. There are multiple different cooling mechanisms the human body has developed, and feet touching a cooler surface is only one of them. It is refreshing to touch the ground with bare feet. Compare this cooling effect with the adverse effect of feet that are covered in shoes with a consistent, elevated temperature pumping into the system from overheated feet.

COLD DAYS

While barefoot running on cold days, your feet may become numb enough that you lose some sensitivity. After a few minutes of the initial discomfort the body will adjust and there is a sense of ease associated with numbed feet. This might sound like it would be distressful, if you haven't experienced it, but it's actually quite comfortable! Using the cold as a trigger to turn on the body's thermal regulation system is a potential bonus benefit. Studies done by a university in the Netherlands, showed that cold temperature triggered positive changes on the immune system. The popularity of some social media stars, who built their stardom popularizing ancient cold weather balancing skills, prove that people viscerally connect to their body's response to cold.

There are other clothing items we should mention, besides shoes. It's troubling to me that I continue to see people run in "plastic" (man-made materials) clothing, sometimes even sweat suits that promote excessive sweating, or just tend to be over-dressed in general. This tends to occur especially when people are trying to lose weight. For some reason people still believe that the weight they lose this way is fat when in fact it is simply water. Over-dressing makes the body lose vital minerals and excessive amounts of water, which is unhealthy for the body, and consequently, it is improbable to achieve a healthy weight-loss under unhealthy circumstances.

Science has discovered that every single cell in the body is in some sort of communication with all the other cells via a form of light communication. Wearing any type of "plastic" clothing inhibits the body to work at its optimal performance because it disrupts this light communication on the cellular level.

Ideally, try wearing the least amount of clothing you can get away with. The more the body's surface is exposed to fresh air the better the body's self-regulating temperature system can work. Clothing also restricts the proper operation of the sweat glands.

People today are dangerously low in Vitamin D, due to the skins lack of an efficient amount of exposure to sun light, which according to research, could be the cause of many illnesses. Exposed skin outdoors is great for triggering Vitamin D production in your body.

Based on the thickness of your thighs you might opt for tights that cover your upper legs to avoid chaffing on longer runs. This is an issue for overweight people and heavily muscular individuals as well. In comparison to what the body weight of a healthy hunter gatherer normally is, we are all somewhat overweight. I certainly feel that I have way too much extra weight on me every time I spend time with real (full time) hunter-gatherers.

Even in colder climates you will want to wear the least amount of clothing you can manage. It's easy to overdress in the cold, but usually once you get moving the body heats up significantly and most of the layers do become unnecessary. Sweating will draw heat from your body and you could end up being much colder than you would be with less clothing. As I mentioned earlier, utilizing the cold weather's positive effects on your body holds some - yet not fully understood- health benefits.

Hats are pretty popular amongst runners. In hotter climates people wear them for protection from the sun, but according to some studies hats are completely a 'take it or leave it' item. The coolness you gain from the shade of the hat is lost due to the lack of air circulation around your head. Without a hat you are more exposed to the sun, but you have the air circulation cooling you.

If you are concerned about the sun, just use a healthy sunscreen lotion and apply it thick. Or, ideally, wear nature's hat and let your hair grow out if you can manage. When you have longer hair, it gives you the protection against the sun and as your hair moves while running, it creates a cooling air flow around your neck and scalp. Nature got it right, again.

The bottom line:

Wear the least amount of clothing you feel you could be comfortable in. Leave your hair down and let it cool your head while at the same time protecting yourself from the sun.

8. ADDITIONAL SURPRISING BENEFITS

Persistence Running is a unique and complicated subject.

It is complicated because our entire existence is intertwined with the subject; we evolved to partake in this method of hunting and therefore it is ingrained in us. When we are so close to something it's often hard to gain perspective on it.

It's also quite a large subject, because everything that resides in you is, in one way or another, a part of and connected to Persistence Running. It would take another book to cover all of its effects on our bodies, so I'm not going to attempt to do it here. I don't believe science and our understanding of the human body is at a level where we can comprehend all that is involved to run the way a human being was built to run.

Science is usually in catch up mode to what specialists and masters of fields already know from experience. I will expand on some recent discoveries in this next chapter, which are great examples of this delay in scientific understanding.

FEELING GOOD

Most people have heard of the 'runner's high', which right up until recently, sports science contributed to elevated dopamine levels. Recently there have been some new discoveries in regards to 'runner's high'. The name actually fits the description more than anyone realized, in regards to what takes place within the human body while someone is running. Science finally learned what all runners have been feeling for a long time! The body releases a cannabis-like chemical while we run longer distances. One of the pleasant side effects of running long distances is that it feels good, like a natural 'high'!

Of course, this 'feel good' effect cannot be an accident. Nature always wisely 'designs' everything in a way that if it's good for your existence, it also feels good to do it. Going to the bathroom to

elieve yourself feels good and it is good for you. Having sexual
ntercourse also feels good, because it is good for your being - it
not only connects you chemically to your partner, but also helps
you to replicate yourself, or at least your DNA, in the form of a
cute baby!

SWEAT

Our bodies were designed with a sophisticated sweat gland system
to aid us in long distance runs in high heat. During the highest
heat, when even cheetahs will sit out a hunt, we have a built-in
cooling system to keep going strong. In fact, it is much easier to
run an animal into the ground with Persistence Running when
temperatures soar over 105 degrees Fahrenheit. Most animals are
either in the shade keeping cool or, if they are moving, they are on
the run from a predator! But they are not able to do both at the
same time.

Nature is a master at creating characteristics that serve multiple
purposes. Another wonderful purpose of sweating profusely
in high heat is that it is also a great cleansing methodology.
Researchers examined every cleansing method known to the
human body, including modern and traditional medicine, looking
to discover what was the most effective way to cleanse the body
of harmful substances. Sweating beat every other method,
exponentially so that there was practically no second place.

Sweating in high heat while running animals down did not only
make the hunt more probable to succeed, but in the process, we
were also able to cleanse our system.

EYE SIGHT

When you run like a Persistence Runner, you must gaze in the
distance. Not only are you following and chasing down something
that is ahead of you, you are doing it in an environment where,
unless you are aware of your surroundings, you might end up
becoming the prey, if you are not careful! Our eyes have a big role
in orientation while tracking, chasing, and running.

Looking into the distance, searching for the animal (or pretending to search for the animal, in our modern world), also has some very positive side effects, this time, for your eyes. Your eyes are controlled by tiny muscles, which are only fully relaxed while you are sleeping or while you are looking into the distance. The closer something is, which you are looking at, the harder those eye muscles need to work to keep the object in focus. As I am writing these words to you, my own eye muscles are working hard so I can keep the letters on the computer screen in focus. In our modern world where we spend so much time indoors, there are no possibilities to gaze into the distance without, literally, hitting a wall. Keeping healthy eyesight for a whole lifetime is almost unheard of. How many people do you know over the age of 43 who don't rely on glasses? Maintaining better eyesight is also one of the potential positive side effects of running long distances as a Persistence Runner.

The pleasant chemicals released during the 'runner's high' effect, the detoxification, and the eyesight conditioning (not to mention plenty of more not so obvious effects of Persistence Running) can improve your experience in life. I am sure science will gradually unfold more and more information about running to prove why and how it feels good, how it leads to better health and why it is necessary for people to live a good, long life!

9. COMPETITION AND OTHER PITFALLS

HOW TO LAST

Now that we've begun to wrap our minds around the perspective of Persistence Running, let's bring some awareness to the potential psychological hazards we might encounter due to the modern sentiments and training methods that circulate.

During the rare occasion when hunter-gatherers' and modern competitions meet, we can witness in their behavior the distinctly unique and different approach to racing. When the Tarahumara Indians entered and won ultra-distance running events in the 90's, they succeeded by following (persistence hunted, basically) the leaders of the race and only close to the finish line did they overtake the frontrunners. This was the only way the Tarahumara could probably make sense of running for a long period of time without substantial meaning and purpose. In my experience and my research involving long distance running tribes, the capability developed for the purpose of hunting to consume animal protein. The long-distance running capability was also potentially used to deliver messages between related tribes to create and maintain good cooperation networks. Based on the San tribe's continuous egalitarian society, competition for the sake of winning doesn't make sense. I once witnessed the brutal teasing of a hunter who took down an animal. At first it seemed very odd, but after further contemplation I realized this way the success of the individual hunter will not disrupt his or her ego, by believing that he or she is better than the others. This very anti-capitalistic thinking is very foreign today for most people in the world. I think I have a little more of a sharp eye for it because I still remember my youth in a socialist society where individual success was not in the center focus. Traditional tribes developed fierce tools to keep a sense of equality amongst all members of the group. Just like we in our western world are aware that too low of a self-esteem could lead to mental illness over time, the traditional tribes also believed that too high of a self-esteem could lead to a different type of negative outcome. Maybe there is a lesson in this for all of us.

Competitions are the means to an end for the human psyche. I have worked with numerous athletes and sport teams that competed at high levels, and eventually everyone burns out. If your goal is to be healthy and exercise for your own well-being, or, if you want to master Persistence Running, you must evaluate where you are in terms of being competitive. Otherwise, you might, literally, run out of fuel prematurely (way before the time your productive life ends).

Runners always want to improve their pace, or run a particular distance faster. Walkers always want to know how many steps they took, and see how well they did comparatively to their last walk.

As soon as the concept of performance shows up in your mind, you will want to think over the following:

Humans did not become the most energy sufficient mammals by wasting energy. We are wired to conserve energy. Any time when you over-do something without a reason embedded into natural survival you are working against your well-being. We only ran when there was a good reason to run. Persistence hunting yielded to such high probability of succeeding and 'winning' large amounts of meat for the tribe, that running hard, but within our capabilities, made evolutionary sense. Other persistence hunter species, for example African wild dogs, have always been ranked as the most successful hunters amongst the large carnivorous members of an ecosystem. Because the state of our general conditioning level is so low in our modern world, it makes sense that running down an animal seems like a super human achievement, but structurally for our bodies -when conditioned properly- it is a fairly easy thing to do. Unlike other hunting techniques, the persistence hunter doesn't need to worry about the direction of the wind or the right hunting circumstances to be present; the hunter can simply spot the prey, run after it, track it, then eventually out-run it. Some research studies compared different styles of hunting methods, which were conducted over a variety of carnivorous species (including human unting techniques, excluding guns and explosives), and persistence unting yielded to the highest success rate across species (interspecies collaboration, for example humans hunting with the id of hunting dogs ranked very high as well). The energy we spent on running came back several folds when we exhausted the animal beyond its capability of recovering, and hence plenty of dinner was out on the table for everyone.

While persistence hunters ran after an animal, they didn't know how long they had to last. A persistence hunter had to be ready to perhaps even run for most of the day! Essentially, you are running a race where you are unaware of the finish line. In this type of 'life or death' race the persistence runners needed to conserve energy and only push themselves as much as it made sense and not a stride more. The tempo of the animal was relevant, but as long as the hunter was able to stay relatively close to its potential prey and scare it off in regularly timed intervals, the hunt was on track towards succeeding. All animals at max speed easily out run a human being, however – luckily for human beings as persistence hunters - animals only run away when they need to and they run only as far as they must to feel safe, and not a stride longer. Running after an animal was not about speed, but about outlasting them, and periodically pushing the animal to switch into a faster pace; humans built their hunt on destroying the animal's recovery capability. The hunters not only had to focus on the animal, but also had to constantly keep a balance between their inner and outer environment, so they didn't run out of energy, overheat, or become the prey of some other animals. Out in the wilderness, running dry, or running out of energy, literally meant death. Human beings could not afford to test their limits; it would have been abnormal in terms of survival. Collapsing after crossing the finish line of a Marathon, or feeling a high level of exhaustion after a race are signs of abnormal levels of imbalance within the body in healthy human performance terms.

Staying together with your tribe during Persistence Hunting was also key, because the other members of the tribe were also reading the tracks and the wiser -probably older- runners with their superior tracking skills were essential in succeeding in the hunt; losing track of an animal equaled complete failure. It was a loss of vital energy with no proper replenishment. The lost track led to a huge waste of effort and energy, which is unwise in terms of survival. Effort with no reward equals weakness; weakness in nature results in being sorted out.

Running in packs -without competition amongst each other- was key to succeed as a Persistence Hunter.

Every time a modern runner speeds up to the level of her or his maximum capability (physically or psychologically) in the process of trying to measure up to an imaginary standard, the runner runs the risk of missing the type of focus she or he is wired to perform, therefore eventually burning out. Even though runners today do not often risk dying by pushing their limits (there is plenty of Gatorade available to save you), they can burn out by not enjoying the run, and on a long enough timeline, that leads to quitting.

If a runner wants to stay a runner and use running as a means to a healthy lifestyle, then she or he needs to keep focusing on the type of running humans are wired to perform and gain experiences that are sustainable for an entire lifetime. It is not enough to extend our lives; we also need to be able to insert quality into those extended years.

This doesn't mean you always have to run super comfortably, but your increased speed needs to come about in human scale as well. Giving it all you've got during a sprint is hardly ever the way a human being has tried to escape anything, because we were always slower in short distances than most animals – even a house cat could hunt you down in short distance. Running faster from time to time, for example when a Persistence Runner rushes towards its prey to scare it, requires elevated speed, but not full out sprinting. Full out sprinting increases the risk of injuries – and also potentially brings too much commotion to the scene. Human hunters always tried to be low profile enough to keep the attention of larger predators away.

10. FOR COMPETITIVE ATHLETES

If you are currently a competitive runner, one day you will have to go through the extremely difficult 'learning how to run without performance', once you have retired. Once the competitive days are over you will not retire from life; you will still want to keep in good health. Many pro athletes don't look very healthy ten years into their retirement. It is hard to motivate one's self once the 'best' performance is not possible anymore. Interestingly, pulling back and switching focus away from performance made some of the best athletes have break throughs in their professional careers, including my colleague, Mark Allen - who won the Hawaiian Ironman World Championship six times in a row and was named the best endurance athlete of all time by ESPN.

The bottom line is: Competition in running or walking was unheard of during the 99.99% of our evolutionary development. This makes it pretty obvious why neither our minds, nor our bodies are able to handle that way of performing for very long, and definitely not for an entire lifetime. Most people burn out with exercising by pushing themselves too far. Listening to our bodies and our minds with the Persistence Running Principles in mind during exercising, while staying away from concerns of speed and pace, are key to ensuring longevity.

11. BREATHING AND SPEED

As I mentioned earlier, while I was going through my base canoeing conditioning, I grew to hate running, because the high levels of expectation led to a competition induced psychological burn out. But that did not mean that my experiences of running three times a week during my formidable years did not bring me any wisdom. The regular struggle, pain and discomfort forced me to understand the importance of breathing. Since I was considered a good runner, even as a youngster, I was often asked by others how they could run better. My answer was always the same: *"There is no pain that won't go away while you are running, as long as you put all of your focus into your breathing."*

The early understanding of different strategies for breathing eventually led me to use breathing as a tool while working with all types of endurance athletes. My early, personal experiences had to be followed by decades of multi-layered education on breathing to connect the dots. Bringing personal experience to the level of

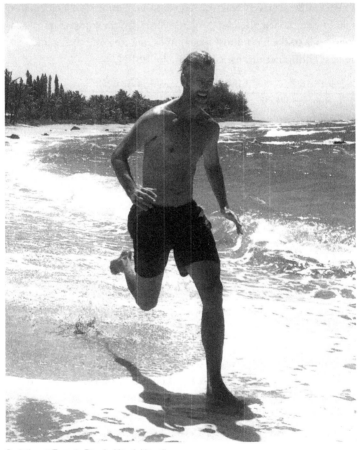

Sprinting at Tunnels Beach, Kauai, Hawaii

conscious awareness is always a necessary step in communicating a useful tool to others as a coach.

There are three (plus one) gears that people have in terms of speed and breathing. I will come to the 'plus one' as the last gear.

Ideally, the most frequently used breathing should be **Nose Breathing** (first gear). I want to emphasize 'ideally' here, because that does not mean Nose Breathing is utilized as much as it should be used even by competitive athletes - let alone the average person moving about. In our modern world, according to related studies, about half of the population breathes through their mouths, mostly. Without the use of complicated descriptions on how human nose breathing works, the basics are what matter the most. When you breathe through your nose your body is encouraged not only to supply your body with oxygen, but also to build energy through your parasympathetic nervous system. Your body either uses up energy with its sympathetic nervous system, or it builds up energy via the parasympathetic nervous system. In practical terms, building energy while using up energy is very useful for a moving body. Generating energy while being active can significantly extend the amount of time one can move without running out of energy. Nose breathing triggers the parasympathetic energy building system of the body.

You are using your first gear when you only breathe through your nostrils; the 'long distance' gear. Extending the capability of utilizing only Nose Breathing even while moving faster will not only increase your endurance capabilities, but will also affect your overall speed in your other 'speed gears'. With Nose Breathing you can even last through extreme ultra- marathon distances. In your daily life, well-utilized nose breathing habits will also lead to multiple other health benefits (including increased blood vessel size, improved sleep quality and improved circadian rhythms, just to mention a few). The scientifically understood benefits of nose breathing are only being fully discovered as we speak, but you might be able to experience them yourself when you practice more nose breathing.

Over a certain level of elevated performance, it does not matter how good your first gear is, you will need to open your mouth to be able to exhale to quickly release a build-up of excess CO_2. This is when you switch into your second gear, **Mixed Breathing**. Using the second gear you are still able to inhale via your nose, but now you must use your mouth for efficient exhalation; this is why I call this the 'Mixed Breathing' speed. This way of breathing has a definite end to it before the body simply cannot continue. With good conditioning methodologies, athletes can improve on their second gear capabilities to manage running even Marathon distances using this more exhausting, but faster speed gear. While you use this type of breathing technique it means you are pushing your system and you are not having a pleasant experience.

Due to the general low level of conditioning of the first gear (Nose Breathing) a surprising amount of people switch into their second gear (Mixed Breathing) even just walking up a set of stairs. Obviously, this is one sign of a majorly de-conditioned state.

A Persistence Runner only switches into this mixed way of breathing on rare occasions - towards the end stages of a hunt.

When you really begin pushing your own capabilities you will switch into **Full Face Breathing**, your third gear. While full face breathing, the nose will not be able to clean the air inhaled via the sophisticated nose-hair cleaning process, however this is not an issue because you will never be able to use this type of breathing for very long. It doesn't matter how much more air you inhale with Full-Face breathing you can only maintain your top speed for a very short period of time. In natural settings it was 'unnatural' to approach maximum speed capacity on a frequent basis. Of course, people always have the capability to condition themselves to do something their bodies were not designed to do - just as you can take your Ferrari out to race on dirt roads, it can do it, but it might not be the wisest idea. At this high-performance level, your being is very exposed to injuries both physically and psychologically. In natural settings people only switched into the third gear (Full Face Breathing) level of performance when they needed to escape from life-threatening situations, or finish off 'jobs' that yielded to a substantial amount of food (energy) intake (for example hunting large animals).

Besides the Nose Breathing, the Mixed Breathing and the Full-Face Breathing there is a plus one gear, the **Breath Withholding**. Lifting up heavy objects and very short, extremely fast activities might require the body to hold breath because even one single breath could destabilize or slow down the system.

Olympic weightlifters know that you must hold your breath in order to lift weights close to your maximum capability. Indeed, some of the body's lifting mechanisms do not work at their maximum capability, unless withholding the breath takes place. With-holding breath is a commonly used weightlifting technique while lifting heavy loads. The body's hydraulic amplifier mechanism brings the most out of the muscles that line up beside the lifter's spine, by cutting off circulation of the lower segment of the spine when contracting the deep abdominal wall and tightening the thoracolumbar fascia. To be less technical, imagine yourself like one of those long balloons that clowns use to make animal figures. When you strongly grip one end of the balloon, the rest of the balloon becomes super erect. Your abdominals play the role of the gripping hand and the muscles along your spine are the erect balloon. If you relax your grip, the balloon gets softer. Short distance sprinters also know that all it takes is one breath to lose their edge, and lose the race.

Needless to say, this particular gear, or way of 'non-breathing', could only be maintained for a few seconds. The only time I recommend to use this non-breathing method for people while exercising, is if the individual is extremely well conditioned, due to the large variety of injuries it could potentially bring on. In my experience, the risks of performing so close to the edge outweigh the tiny extra advantage an athlete could gain from exercising at this level. After all, the most successful athletes are the ones who do not get injured and gradually keep getting better. An injured athlete can easily get thrown off track for several weeks from pushing such limits. There are no upsides for the weekend warrior to use this level of performance. One can have a healthy and high-quality life without ever using this capability, in my experience.

The bottom line is: Breath and speed are connected. Learning to focus on the breathing will help you find the speed of your activity without needing to rely on heart rate monitors, lactate testing or even timers.

One last note on breathing:

It is no accident that breathing is the center focus of many meditation techniques. The first Tantric Meditation technique is called Buddha Breathing, because supposedly Buddha reached enlightenment while using a particular breathing method. Many runners enjoy using this kind of focus on breathing while running. I even manage to close my eyes for extended periods of time to meditate while running at the same time; relying on seeing with my bare feet only.

The **Buddha Running** goes as follows: track the incoming air from the moment the breath enters your nostrils and follow it all the way down into the depths of your lungs. Once the breath is at the deepest point, release the focus on the breath and only refocus again when the next inhalation starts. Running this way can become not only a physical activity, but a fully meditative activity as well, which might serve you on multiple levels. It is not the only way to make running into a meditative activity, it is one of the ways; the Buddha breathing way.

12. FOOT LANDING
LANDING SOFTLY

When I consult with people who are well versed in the subject of running, including professional running coaches, they are always the most interested in foot landing. Most running enthusiasts are convinced that there is a 'right way' of landing with the foot and a 'wrong way' of landing.

Any one type of landing that is overused is going to be the 'wrong landing' and every landing can be the 'right landing' on a given surface in a given moment.

As the proprioceptors on the sole of the foot send the message to the brain in regards to what type of surface the foot has landed upon, the brain sends a very specific movement sequence to the body on how to land the foot and how to adjust the body, accordingly.

The combinations of foot landing and body positioning are endless, so giving advice to anyone is just hopeless posturing.

The good news is that if you can manage to take your shoes off, you can trust that your 'body-mind' will take care of it all properly. I love calling this the 'mind-sole' connection, which also ends up feeding your 'soul'.

To be able to move from point A to point B was obviously very important during our evolutionary development. Any genetic lineages that did not have this aspect of physicality perfected have been sorted through the natural selection process.

You have what it takes to move and run very capably: a human brain and physical structure, and a pair of bare feet. Every other part in between will fall into place just fine as long as you don't try controlling the body too much.

This doesn't mean you cannot improve on yourself, as long as you keep the main guidelines in your neocortex (in your conscious mind), while aiming for better overall health.

A Mexican Indian saying goes like this: "When you run on the earth and run with the earth, you can run forever."

The observation of the feet is the best avenue towards self-improvement when it comes to running. The key word is 'observation' and NOT the control of the feet. Let the feet move and land the way it feels the best and observe what that is, as opposed to trying consciously to control a way of landing that you believe you should be using, in terms of proper running. Your conscious mind has major limitations when it comes to affecting fast activities, therefore when you attempt to use the conscious mind to control your landing while running (or even walking) you are asking your conscious mind to perform a task it is simply not equipped to do. The subconscious mind will give the proper instructions to your body on how to land and what length of stride to choose, based on the surface you are on. The conscious mind is only able to potentially observe this lightning-fast continuous adjustment of your body. The observation will serve as an educational tool for you to learn how your body moves naturally. This observation will keep you focused on the present moment wonderfully - and creating yet again another chance to make running into a meditative activity.

The kind of landing one should be aware of while running barefoot is an interesting conversation. It becomes even more interesting when someone has some experience with barefoot running, and barefoot exercising.

The foot can hit hard when speeding on a soft surface, the foot can grab the ground when the ground contains sharp rocks or loose soil and the foot can also be placed gently while landing at any speed over most surfaces.

A hard-hitting foot is what most people know. You've probably witnessed people running downhill making a lot of noise with their feet as they pound the ground. These folks hit the ground hard because the shoes protect their skin. Hitting the foot hard into the ground would never happen while barefoot (unless the ground is very soft; for example, sand).

When running with shoes the skin of the foot is spared from a hard landing (besides some potential blisters from the shoes, which is a regular annoyance for most runners), but the resonation of the hard hit on the ground still needs to go somewhere. The shoes behave like boxing gloves. To anyone who has never boxed before, the boxing glove probably seems like protection. Statistically, the story looks different though, because in fact boxers who fight with thick gloves have significantly more brain injuries than bareknuckle fighters. It's the same reason American football players suffer from such serious injuries, verses rugby players, who also play a very similar game with little to no protection.

When you have no protection, you must be more mindful of your body. That does not mean a rugby player does not hit hard, but they hit with a force their bodies can handle, given the situation, as opposed to an American football player hitting harder than their body can handle due to the body armor, which can result in lifelong injuries of the brain, for example.

Running with shoes will allow the feet to pound the ground much harder than the body was designed to handle. The excessive pounding on the ground forces the body to operate under very stressful circumstances. Though the body will try to lead those excessive forces away from the feet, such adjustments will come with the creation of unnatural stabilization methodologies for

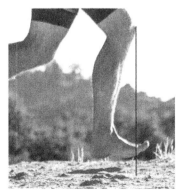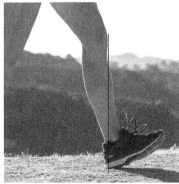

The landing is very different barefoot vs shoed foot

the joints to cope with the pounding. The most obvious of these adjustments are easily noticeable at the knees, because "shoed" runners keep their knees much straighter while running. Barefoot runners discover that eventually their knees bend significantly more (most noticeably perhaps while running downhill) and act as major shock-absorbers, as opposed to being partially locked like shoed runners. In my experience, the reason people keep a straighter knee while running in shoes is because the force with which they allow their feet to hit the ground, would make their knees buckle. The bent knee creates extra cushion and spring for the body and allows the ankle to operate significantly better as well.

LANDING TYPES

The most frequently used landing while barefoot is the **Whole Foot Landing** for all intermediate and advanced runners – beginners learn this during the beginner phase naturally. This is when the entire foot lands at the same time. Though for most "shoed" running enthusiasts this sounds odd, because this is a difficult movement to produce with shoes on. This type of landing is hard to achieve unless the knees are properly freed up. It does make sense to land the foot this way, because the more evenly the weight distribution is spread, the less pressure hits any particular section of the foot; the pressure is being distributed.

The bare foot always lands somewhat like when you speed along with a skateboard and you continuously propel yourself forward with one leg. Before touching the ground with the foot of the propelling leg, the speed of the skateboard is assessed and the positioning of the leg as it touches the ground, aided by a pulling motion, minimizes the friction between the skater's foot and the ground, avoiding a hard hit.

Running barefoot naturally encourages the same type of no-friction landing. Shoe bearing runners hit the ground hard without the appropriate pulling action, overusing their quadriceps relatively to their hamstrings and buttocks. The sense of being pulled forward by the leg is the result of touching and pulling the body forward with the barefoot for the sake of minimizing potentially painful friction between the foot and the ground.

The slightly inward tilted foot landing starts with the touch down of the outer edge of the foot (around the 3rd and 4th metatarsals) and it follows immediately by a gripping motion of the toes. This landing style, which first shows up for intermediate runners, is utilized on a 'sharp' surface (for example little rocks scattered on a soft surface). I call this landing the **Edge Gripping Landing**. Beginners' feet are not able to produce this movement yet. In fact, the sign of intermediate capability for a barefoot practitioner is that naturally they begin to grip this way. Advanced runners have significantly less discomfort on odd surfaces therefore they do not use this type of landing frequently. Advanced barefoot runners also grip with their feet on different types of surfaces - especially on loose soil, slippery surfaces or when running uphill.

The **Heal Strike Landing** is the most frequently used landing for shoed runners. Heal Strike Landing also happens barefooted, but only on deep sand or on soft grass. Whenever the brain instructs you to land that way, do not shy away from it and follow your 'head'.

Mid-foot Landing is regarded as the ideal foot landing for shoed runners. The landing takes place on the front padding of the foot.

This landing pattern, however, for barefoot running, doesn't happen as often because landing with the entire foot allows the body to engage better, though at the acceleration phase a mid-foot landing is often observed.

Front-Foot Landing is used by both shoed sprinters and also by barefoot sprinters. To be able to run this way on any surface barefoot requires an extremely well-conditioned foot, otherwise it is very easy to bruise or fracture the metatarsals in the feet. As a beginner or even intermediate barefoot runner one should stay away from sprinting on harder surfaces and only do it on extremely soft surfaces (for example: deep sand on the beach, or on thicker, soft grass). Though a beginner or intermediate runner might catch themselves using this landing pattern, hopping around certain obstacles while running, they should stay away from using this pattern for longer than a few steps. The description of front foot landing is very similar to the mid-foot landing because the foot lands on the front padding of the foot, but the involvement of the toes is more prominent, due to the high activation of the hamstrings while speeding. This results in the pulling of the torso forward, over the legs. I would like to emphasize that understanding how to land the foot is not very important for an advanced barefoot runner, because at this stage the runner should have a superbly well-conditioned body to handle anything.

While barefoot running, the body often switches from one type of landing to another, frequently, and seamlessly. It really is a marvel how the human brain can swiftly change how the body operates based on what is underneath the foot during any given landing moment.

Most people shy away from running on wet or muddy ground. Surprisingly, running on such ground is very comfortable and enjoyable. While learning about Persistence Hunting from the San tribe in Africa, I found out that the best time to attempt Persistence Hunting is when the first rains arrive after the dry season. Due to the rain, the ground becomes very soft and the animal's hooves sink, while people's duck-like feet stay afloat better on the muddy ground. Running down animals is significantly easier and faster on such wet ground. Once this understanding became clear to me, the extreme comfort I experienced while running in rain was not so surprising anymore; we just might be wired to run best on soggy ground.

The most important aspect of foot landing is surprising to most. Do not attempt to run with a specific landing pattern, nor try to control how your feet land! For the very first section on this new adventure of 'going barefoot' you should observe how genius your own body truly is. Observe your natural landing while you are a beginner, continue the observation while you become an intermediate runner and welcome the predictable landing patterns as you grow wiser in 'reading' the ground with your feet, and your eyes. Once you are experienced enough, you will understand that even the color of the ground –yellow, brown or gray- in different temperatures makes your foot land differently. You will be able to adjust your planned path as a barefoot runner. You will feel as if you have become one with your environment, you run 'with earth' and see with your feet.

13. THE UNITY OF THE BODY PARTS

The human body works as a unit. The feet, calves, quads, buttocks or any of the rest of the body cannot be viewed as an independent unit, when it comes to the human movement. Whenever there is a restriction in one part of the body, it will affect the rest, like a chain reaction. The body will begin making adjustments to compensate, and as a result, it will begin to move differently. Restriction of the foot (due to shoe usage) affects the movement and functions of multiple aspects of the body. Once the foot is freed up it results in changes throughout the entire body.

A transitional phase must take place from the moment the restricted body part moves freely until the newly freed section and the rest of the body synchronize. Bringing awareness to the potential challenges one should look out for while transitioning to shoeless existence is not only useful, but it is also important.

KNEES, HIPS, MOUNTAINS

I've always thought about what the knees full capability is when it comes to running, as it's a hot spot for injuries for most runners who wear ultra-cushioned shoes. My questions were answered once I started to run full-time as a barefoot athlete. The level of force the body pushes into the ground while the feet are wearing shoes is too great to have any knee flexion present.

While running barefoot, the level of knee flexion - the bending of the knee- greatly depends on the incline, or, decline of the path.

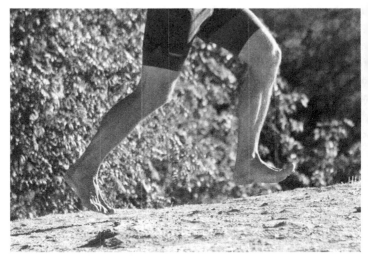

Uphill running and dorsi flexing the foot, tightens the Achilles tendon

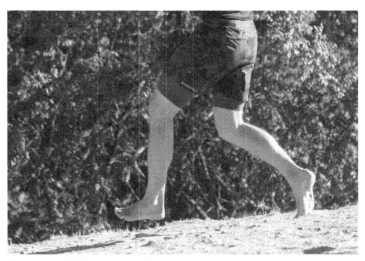

'Cartoon free-falling' running downhill

The more tilted the environment the more the knee is utilized. It is surprising, while running down a steep hill, how much the knees motion resembles a partial squatting position. The heaviness of the runner's steps changes with the varying angles of the ground as well. The steeper the hill the less the runner attempts to fully land in a traditional way. The downhill barefoot landing resembles rather a skimming motion of the ground. This skimming motion of the soles of the feet results in picking up significant pace, utilizing gravity. Often times, barefoot runners report feeling like a cartoon character, barely touching the ground and a feeling of 'free-falling' while gliding downhill.

Uphill, there is an interesting technique I discovered that comes handy to bring more bounce into the running steps. While uphill running pulls the ankle into a forced dorsi flexion (tilting up your foot), this brings about an extra bounce from the Achilles tendon - because as soon as you touch the ground the tendon is already pulled tight. Once someone masters running uphill, the speed and the bounce the runner can produce in the mountains is game changing. If a runner wants to improve his hill running capabilities, this technique is something to test out!

The angle of the runners' pelvis changes with the incline or the decline of the path as well. The pelvis always aims to stay horizontal, which makes sense because our bodies evolved in an area where 'mountain running' was not part of our skill set. Homo Sapiens evolved in a rather flat area, around the Kalahari Desert, where our pelvis would be able to easily keep the horizontal position. Of course, at a certain ground incline or decline this cannot be maintained while running.

The natural question that might arise, given this idea of the maintained pelvic level, is if people should run at all on steep inclines or declines. A hunter-gatherer most possibly switches into a walk in a challenging mountain environment, given the build of the human body. It is probably not beneficial to 'push' the body -from an evolutionary stand point- where the potential for injury increases significantly. Every creature specializes for a particular environment during its evolution. A chimpanzee is specialized in climbing rather than running; this does not necessarily mean it cannot perform running, but overexposure to running would create problems in their joints. Humans are specialized in running long distances on vast open fields, not in the mountains. This point must be kept in mind in the case someone is aiming to be able to run during his or her entire life. This statement is a hard one for me to write down here, because I personally love running in beautiful Alpine environments, but remembering how and where we evolved is a prerequisite for developing and keeping a healthy and capable body.

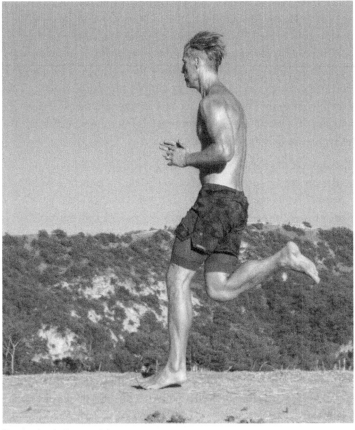

Running free in the mountains

ARMS AND WRISTS

The arms are interesting balancing devices for the walking and the running body. The most basic aspect of the arms' job while running is that the arm needs to move in perfect synchronicity with the opposite leg; a reptilian pattern. When we examine people, this reptilian pattern is often somewhat off by the time someone reaches adulthood, after living in a modern environment. Even slightly out of sync movement between the arms and the legs adds up overtime while running or walking, putting stress onto a series of joints throughout the entire body.

I frequently use some infant development exercises, which are helpful in cleaning up these little understood, but important patterns. Using the body sub-optimally with non-ideal repetitious movements, leads to joint irritations overtime, which are difficult to correct once they occur. These aches and pains show up slowly and leave people wondering what they did to be in pain. But the matter of the fact is that using the left and the right side of the body in a less than optimal way will lead to premature wear-down of the spine, shoulders, hips, knees and ankles.

The arms can move in a straight line back and forth on short, fast, high paced runs (for example a sprint), but mostly the arms move diagonally with the fingers passing slightly through the center line of the body.

While keeping the hands slightly open, you give yet another opportunity to your body to cool itself. The flicking of the wrist provides a small, but noticeable bounce into the next running stride as well. I am aware that the amount of extra movement the flicking of a wrist can give a runner might seem insignificant, but on longer distances anything helps to be more comfortable, and being more energy efficient is useful. The lack of efficient use of any one body part will make some other body parts work harder than they were 'designed' to do. Much of the research done by Harvard Anthropology Professor Daniel Lieberman, points to the speculation that given the right temperature and environment, human beings evolved to be the most capable and energy efficient land mammals on the planet when it come to endurance performance, so we might as well use everything we have to live up to our purpose.

ELBOWS AND SHOULDERS

The movement of the elbow in combination with the shoulders is also an interesting place for discovery. Most of the time people run swinging their arms back and forth, and that is one way of keeping the body balanced while moving. But you may have noticed that even shoe wearing runners, trying to catch their balance while running downhill at a faster pace, move their arms opposite to their usual arm pattern. To visualize this arm pattern, just imagine someone running downhill and almost falling, at which point they would be moving their arms not back and forth, but rather in a forward circular motion (i.e., falling forward arm pattern).

Perhaps the easiest way to understand how to experiment with this is if you imagine you are a steam train and your arms move in a circular pattern as if they are train wheels moving forward.

When you run downhill, or on rough surfaces or simply when you want to have a faster pace, using this forward circling elbow movement will give you some extra swing into your steps and provide better balance. The arm movement reminds me somewhat of a scaled down version of Phoebe Buffet's running pattern in the 'Friends' episode where she goes running with Rachel, if you know the reference (I promise this is my only note in the book that will serves as a pop culture reference point)!

There is no one, two, three or four ways of running, but the combinations of how the feet, ankles, knees, hips, lower back, elbows, and wrists move are countless, based on the degree of the incline, the type of surface and the speed. Purposefully I have left the spine out of this chapter, because the spine requires some extra attention and I will address it in the next chapter.

SPINE

At this point you will not be surprised to know that the spine also moves differently from "shoe" to barefoot activities. The inner environment of the body will always adjust to the outer environment in many ways - as long as there is the proper connection between the environment and the runner. Epigenetics can be observed viscerally by every single one of us when we learn barefoot running, because the outer environment clearly adjusts what happens inside of us. Barefoot running is the proper conduit between the body's inner and outer environment; there is no separation from rubber soles numbing the connection.

The spine is essentially a spring. It is shaped like a traditional bow before the string bends it. The beautiful S shape provides flexibility, spring power and mechanical potential.

The entire body is wrapped around the spine; therefore, it is no surprise that the way the spine acts will significantly affect the movement of all the other body parts; and of course, vice versa. There are plenty of studies found conclusively that lower back discomfort can be managed much better once the individual spends an elevated amount of active time barefooted. The foot creates the base for the active structure and the spine is the core of the structure. The interaction between the two is profound, and in my opinion, not yet understood exactly, but can be felt with practice and focused attention.

As we evolve from physically incapable newborns to capable adults, we go through predictable stages of development. Pretty much anyone who has been around kids knows that a newborn first starts to wiggle from one spot to another. This little wiggling motion is an important step in teaching the spinal structure how to generate force. This little movement eventually becomes more prominent and, once the spine is strong enough, the baby learns how to turn on to the tummy. Step by step, the baby goes through all the stages of learning to move its body. In a natural setting a human being would keep practicing and using these development type movements during their entire life (for example: crawling during a hunt while trying to get closer to the prey).

Unfortunately, in our modern world, many of these developmental movements are not practiced anymore after early childhood - you would even be looked at as a mentally unstable person if you crawled around on your hands and knees.

But the force generating capability of the spine that you gained as a child, must be conditioned regularly in order to keep it throughout your entire life. When analyzing people, I often see that their spine is not efficient in generating force required to run properly. Many injuries to the ankles, knees, hips, shoulders and even the elbows can originate from these areas having to work much harder while trying to make up for the lack of force generated by the spine.
In the *'Exercise Description'* section I will include the 'Inch Worm' exercise (basically the wiggling I mentioned above), which can help to recondition some lost force generating capabilities of the spine.

The interaction of the feet, that have the contact with the surface your body is moving upon, and the spine that is generating much of the force by angulating and rotating, is a relationship you will be able to sense more and more as your barefoot capabilities improve. The micro rotation of the foot caused by the spines' rigidity doesn't hurt, or may not be felt, in shoes (you might wear down the bottom of your shoes faster). While you are barefoot, these micro rotations may be felt and cause discomfort. The body always moves away from pain and -in my experience- the spine is encouraged to move more to decrease this discomfort.

LOWER BACK

The position of the lower back will change based on the incline or decline of the surface and the speed of the individual. There is also a continuous angulation of the spine that happens while moving. This angulation ideally provides a momentum to the body to move forward efficiently, utilizing all available elastic and muscular energy in the body.

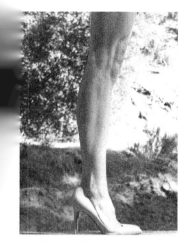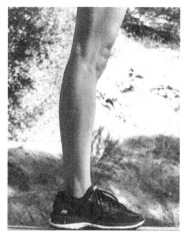

The alignment of the leg is similar when the heel is elevated in high-heeled shoes or thick heeled shoes

When it comes to running shoes, companies attempt to soften the negative effects of a drastic heal strike by building sophisticated structures into a shoe. These structures really confuse the entire body and throw the entire system out of balance. Even a slightly elevated heal will create significant changes in how the spine (usually the lower back) curves or how the knee behaves.

An altered lower back position will result in hip and pelvic tilt changes. These hip changes can rotate the legs inwards. Adjusting the knees natural position (creating a semi-locked knee position) and forcing the ankles to behave differently often times lead to hyper mobility at the ankles and lack of mobility at the knees. Of course, the extra degree added to the curve in the lower back also effects the mid-back and the neck position. Running in high heels is a goofy idea by anyone's standards, but thick healed running shoes are comparable to lower 'high heels' - from the view point of how the lowerback's position changes.

While you stand barefoot your lower back position will probably be somewhat different from when you are wearing shoes. While you are moving barefoot the difference between the movement of the lower back and all collaborating joints will be drastically different as well. Information of these changes can easily be found these days from resources ranging from the Harvard Skeletal Lab to the American College of Rheumatology, and many more.

MIDDLE & UPPER SPINE

As the mobile upper back moves back and forth, the gained momentum provides an extra bounce in the body as it moves forward. There is a rhythm that must take place for the runner to be able to access this extra bounce, which is very sensitive to the body's positioning. This rhythm is much easier to learn barefoot than with shoes on, because there is much more information available for your brain to gather to be able to guide the body while you are barefoot.

The very top of the spine, the neck or cervical spine area, also does its job, but it is more focused on the stability of the head instead of aiding into the 'swing' of the momentum. I have seen fatigued shoe runners running with their heads bobbing from side to side. When a critical structure -such as the head- is not balanced while running, it is a sign that the runner's body is out of sync with the demands of the mind. Bobbing the head from side to side is something I have never seen anyone able to do while running barefoot. A natural surface in my definition is a surface that is constantly changing. It is very possible to run on unnatural surfaces, for example asphalt or track, but those surfaces will act as a shoe, in some perspective, since they provide no changing environment for the foot and the body. Interestingly, a not well-maintained asphalt road can sometimes provide enough variety to the brain to have a 'good' running experience without overusing any one part of the foot.

With the right base and connection provided by the foot between the ground and the body, the spine will bend, rotate and angulate resulting in plenty of energy from the core to initiate a wave, which will end up as the full spectrum movement of the human body.

14. STRETCHING & MASSAGING

Will I need to stretch in the same way if I run barefoot as opposed to running with shoes? This is a question I receive regularly.

To address flexibility in its entirety would require me to write multiple books, but I am going to touch on the more 'grounded' ideas on stretching as part of this handbook.

In a natural habitat no creatures need to stretch in ways that people in the modern world understand stretching. A natural human habitat would be the environment emulating the life of a hunter-gatherer in the area of the Kalahari-Okavango Delta in modern day Botswana/Namibia in Africa.

We can witness the natural 'stretching' of a balanced creature when we observe a leopard or a chimpanzee stretching after waking up from sleep. People still stretch this way as well, but for a person living in a modern (restrictive) environment, this type of stretching would not be enough to keep all joints properly mobile. Due to the lack of variety in people's movements and activities in their days, months, seasons and years, many aspects of people's bodies are neglected and 'stiffen' up over time.

It is possible to live perfectly in the modern world, but it is not easy. Unless someone can manage to bring in enough walking, running, climbing, tossing, pulling, pushing, jumping, chopping, crawling, and hanging into their lives, people must supplement their bodies with extra mobilization, including stretching activities. These activities are part of a corrective procedure to keep the body well balanced in an unnatural habitat. For more comprehensive information on the subject, please look out for my upcoming book on Core Survival Ability Benefitting Activities (C.S.A.B.A.).

There is a correlation between the decreased need for stretching when someone starts running (or even spending more time) barefoot. The body will move less predictably -in always changing patterns- as opposed to responding to the environment monotonously. There will be less overuse of one particular way of moving. The larger variety of movement will not allow the feet, ankles, knees, and hips to stiffen up due to the repetitive movement - especially during longer distances.

Of course, unless you have a complete balanced running regiment with a variety of seasons (ultra-distance runs, speedy & steady tempo runs, sprints, running drills, walks, hikes, etc.) in your life, you will still need to stretch even as a barefoot runner or walker.

In the 'Practical Stretching' section, please find our general, but full, running related stretching routine. Frequent practice of these stretches will improve your chances to keep all of your joints mobile and establish a better range of motion around your joints.

15. EXTRA CONDITIONING EXERCISES

HOW LONG WILL IT TAKE?

Extra conditioning is not an absolute necessity, because being barefoot will only let you do as much as your feet's current condition allows you to do. But I am aware that there are runners who want to speed up the process, because going from a shoe runner to a barefoot runner takes a considerable amount of time to adjust.

There are some activities one can do to somewhat speed up the improvement and development as a barefoot runner.

If you've lived your life in shoes your feet are de-conditioned and deformed, relatively to the rest of your body. Doing some extra conditioning to bring the feet up to the condition of the rest of your body might be wise.

It is hard to estimate exactly how long it takes for anyone to make the transition, but here is a general guideline.

If you are an *experienced runner* with no significant injuries, and you switch to full-time barefoot running, it will take you approximately one year and a half to work yourself back up to your current "shoe-ed" capability level of running. This does not mean you are going backwards during that time. Often times runners who switch over to barefoot running test their running skills from time to time by putting on their old shoes. Over all they can experience speed improvement, but often feel awkward and eager to take off their shoes as soon as possible.

If you are not a well-conditioned runner and you are interested in starting barefoot conditioning, you are probably going to enjoy the process more – no frustrating expectations. It will not take longer to condition yourself barefoot in comparison to shoed conditioning – just without risking long term discomforts and injuries.

You will also probably not be concerned about breaking previous addictions regarding speed, pace, distances and times for running. The attention you receive from fellow runners due to being barefoot will give you loads of encouragement, so you will probably not be concerned about improving your capabilities in traditional terms. Most likely, you will be a lone warrior as a 'barefooter' in your area. I believe barefoot running and walking will have a comeback, because it makes sense; it feels good and resonates true to the practitioners once they pass the initial fear of taking their shoes off.

SOME PRACTICAL EXERCISES

In the case you want to speed up the improvement of your pace, I do have good news for you. Some great running cultures have traditions they practice that result in more robust bone density in their bodies. You can also practice these ritualistic traditions in your life as supplementary activities (exercises).

The African Maasai people jump up and down around fires, sometimes for hours, as a ceremonial activity. During these ceremonies they fall into a trance and have visions. You do not need to go to the great lengths of reaching a trance, but if you jump up and down regularly on a hard, natural surface, and gradually increase the amount of time you spend on this activity, you will be able to improve an important aspect of your running tool - the bone density in the bones of your feet. As a side effect you might also discover a new meditative movement, which could serve you in multiple different ways - just as meditation does. See the description of the '**Maasai Jumping**' in the *'Exercise Description'* section.

A very different culture, the communist Soviet sport conditioning system, also created robust bone structures for their sprinters. The Soviet sprinting coaches made athletes jump onto concrete, barefoot, from ladder steps, gradually moving higher and higher up. It is a rather brutal sounding way of conditioning athletes, but in fact it is a compact and effective way of reaching results relatively fast as long as you use common sense, don't push the boundaries, and take your time. The danger in this technique is doing too much too soon. You will need to make sure to be very careful in increasing the height of the ladder slowly. There is nothing to lose by being slower in increasing the take-off height, but there is a lot to lose in being too fast. See the description of the '**Soviet Ladder**' exercise in the *'Exercise Description'* section.

Improving the energy generating capability of the spine also brings a tremendous amount of upside within itself. You can mimic a four-month-old baby's movements to improve/refresh this capability of your spine. At around this age, a baby is working on the 'wiring' and strengthening of all the muscles around her or his spine. Via this infant development movement, the baby becomes agile enough that they can travel little distances by simply using their spine to '**inch worm**' them from point A to point B.

Under natural circumstances this 'inch worm' movement capability is meant to improve throughout a versatile and mobile life. In modern life, beyond early childhood, most people lose tremendous capabilities in regards to their spine's force output. This is a safe exercise to practice, because it is almost impossible to over-do it. The first task for most people is to actually be able to perform the movement. Later the goal becomes to increase the precision of the exercise. Once there is precision in place, the endurance capability eeds to be addressed in the 'inch worming' capability of the spine. ee the description of the '**Inch Worm**' exercise in the *'Exercise Description'* section.

There are plenty of traditional 'gym' exercises one can do to aid n barefoot running (or walking) capabilities, but perhaps nothing provides as good of a base conditioning as becoming great at unging. Primordial movement patterns are the most basic elements of any complex action the human body can produce. For example: when you throw a javelin, you use the pushing pattern with your arm, the rotational pattern with your spine and the lunging pattern with your legs.

Lunges are a great way to improve your muscular strength and endurance in a way that your body can transfer it into running. On some of my journeys I managed to examine how incredible hunter-gatherers were in the lunging primordial movement pattern*. Traditionally raised hunter-gatherers can perform, with relative ease, approximately 150 lunges on each side before they report noticeable fatigue. Most people who have performed lunges before will understand that this is a high number of lunges. I always set out for all of my clients to be able to match at least this number of lunges as part of their general conditioning in preparation to becoming barefoot runners. See the description of the '**Lunges**' exercise in the *'Exercise Description'* section.

I always recommend to people to engage with skilled coaches, to guide them in furthering their capabilities in any exercise. The problem I encounter in referrals, when it comes to barefoot conditioning, is that there are only very few coaches with experience to actually help people. The lack of available coaching was the main motivation in writing this short handbook, to be able to create a guiding aid for people on their barefoot journey.

I encourage you to reach out to us for tips, ideas or simply just to join the community at www.coachbarefoot.com.

Lunges are part of the six primordial patterns, along with squatting, bending, pulling, pushing and rotating, which provide a base to all other more complicated movements the body can produce.

16. HAZARDS & SIGNS

Yes, there are hazards to being barefoot. The hazards that most people are concerned about, before they start their barefoot journey, are not the real hazards.

The process of cleaning your feet with more attention after each barefoot run will not only remove the dirt from your feet, but will also bring a new appreciation towards your feet. And as far as skin related infections go, statistically they decrease as someone spends more time barefoot.

The true hazards lie in pushing yourself beyond your capabilities. Most of the time though your body will give you signs before you can cause any serious harm to yourself.

HEAT

If you live in an area where the weather turns very hot you will need to be cautious of the times when you are outside barefoot. On the hottest days of the summer when the temperatures soar into the hundreds, it can be painful to be on darker surfaces. Your feet can blister up in a matter of minutes. In my experience, everyone runs into one or two situations that bring awareness to limitations when it comes to heat. As you become more advanced in barefoot activities your feet will be able to handle much more, but it is a process. Since you will still spend a large amount of time in shoes, even if you would switch 100% to barefoot exercising, most likely you still wouldn't have the capacity to handle heat over 105 degrees, but that's not a problem. There is no extra benefit in running in heat that high in our modern world. I am writing this book for people who are interested in adapting to the environment we evolved to exist in and not for those who are trying to go back to the ancient ways; that will be a different book, someone else will have to write.

So, when it is hot out, try to go running early in the morning or late in the evening, and have some Luna Sandals or Vibram Five Fingers in your backpack as an emergency backup.

DULL PAINS

Once you have begun garnering some good capabilities and you are charged up from your own improvements, make sure not to ignore dull pains and aches. Rather give yourself an extra couple of days to heal up perfectly from bruises on the feet than push yourself unnecessarily into further injury. I actually never came across anyone who injured themselves while doing barefoot running conditioning. This note is more for the people who use shoes as well in some percentage of their process; for example, Vibram Five Fingers. A little dull pain one day can grow into a broken metatarsal if it is pushed too hard with Five Fingers or minimalist shoes.

BURN OUT

And then there is the mental burn out. Enjoying the process is a prerequisite to improvement and for longevity, in any activity – not only in running. If you are not careful and you frequently push your maximum capabilities, you will burn out and stop. I keep the principle of 'finishing on a high' with every session as a very important priority to keep in mind.

People can experience activities in one way, and later remember the same situation in a completely different way. The way the finish, or completion of an activity is experienced, leaves a much deeper, long lasting imprint in your memory. If you are always deeply exhausted at the end of an exercise session, or cannot wait to finish with it, because you are in some sort of pain, you will have a hard time coming back to 'get more'.

Finishing on a high note by slowing down if you are in pain, switching to walking from running, or even stopping to enjoy nature, will leave a good last impression of your session. At the end of a session, find a way to focus on the positive aspect of it, so your mind can develop a memory you want to recreate the next time.

Our ancestors had it easy in these regards, because Persistence Hunting yielded to an 80% success rate, and that meant at the end of a persistence run they had a huge reward: a massive feast. Our persistence running ancestors always had amazing memories of running long distances, because the big energy output led to an even larger energy intake. It will take a while before you can run with the goal of running down a kudu or some other large antelope, so in the meantime, remember to design - somewhat artificially- those nice, positive experiences at the end of each session! Sometimes this is an easy task and sometimes you will need to be creative.

Always keep a balance between your physicality and your psyche, because you will need both if you want to enjoy the 'active lifestyle' for the rest of your life.

17. DUALITY IN RECOVERY

There is a duality that exists in improving your capabilities in anything in life and this is particularly true when it comes to barefoot running and exercising.

To be able to do well in activities you also need to do well in resting. Rest hard so you can train hard.

Hitting the ground with a relatively relaxed and soft foot is important so the foot can easily mold to the ground it lands on, with each step. But at the moment of touch down, the softness of the foot must switch quickly into a taut firmness to be able to bounce you into your next step effectively. Let go and relax your body between each step so you can use the bouncing effect of the rhythmical muscular contraction from each step.

The only way the body can continuously come back and develop more capabilities is if it has an appropriate amount of time to recover, plus build back some extra capabilities from the last time. People often keep doing and doing without adequate recovery; a process that leads to overtraining. You can only work hard as long as you know how to rest hard, not only between each work out, but even between two steps.

FOLLOWING NATURE'S CLOCK

Traditionally, when people lived according to nature's clock, once the sun set, people's sleep hormones made them relax and prepare to rest. Midday, when the sun past over its zenith, people moved into the shade to have a midday rest. Following nature's clock, people did not waste energy, and were able to live with balanced recovery times after an environmental, social or chemical stressor.

Today, most people stay up way too late and, according to the Harvard Medical School, compelling evidence suggests that one of the prominent (based on my experience the most prominent) reasons why people become sick, drained, overweight, and unhappy on massive scales. This statement might surprise you at first, but without a proper bed time, without proper quality and amount of sleep, your body will go into a consistent stress cycle mode. This will shut down -at least in part- your digestive system, reproductive system, and mess with all organ's circadian rhythms. It will alter hormone levels, and the body will not be able to properly rebuild what was used up from the previous day. Under stress the body 'hangs onto' energy, preparing for lean times – which is useful for a hunter-gatherer, but it only means weight gain for someone who lives in the modern world.

Mind the natural cycles that exist around you and put as much (if not more) importance on resting as you put into doing. Stressors in your life add up. A new and interesting job is a good stressor, an argument on the street for a parking spot is a bad stressor. All stressors (good and bad), though, add up in the day.

Take into consideration that when multiple new events are happening in your life, or, when you are busy, try going to sleep as early as possible - ideally by 9 pm, the latest. If you are having a relatively normal period in your life, you might be able to get away with going to sleep as late as 10:30 pm. But you will never be able to fully recover if you go to sleep later than 10:30 pm on the long haul. People do not realize that their physical recuperation period does not start when they decide to go to sleep but happens throughout the entire night. The decision to sleep is only one of the necessary factors in recovery; it also needs to happen at the right time of the evening. If you are not asleep at the time when you were designed to go to sleep, you will miss out on the chance to fully recover. A generally little known - but well researched - sleep fact is that physical recuperation mostly takes place between 10 pm and 2 am. Going to sleep is supposed to take place in the evening (starting at 10 pm) of the time zone you are most accustomed to. If you go to sleep at 11 pm, for example, you will be missing out on at least one hour from the four-hour physical recuperation phase of that night's sleep. That is a 25% loss of physical recuperation from that particular day. Missing out regularly on recuperation will not only destroy your quality experience in life, but also age you faster. What you cannot build back up will stay used up; a used up human being is an aging human being. We all know very youthful elderlies and very old 30-year-olds. Aging is more optional than most people realize. In nature people age drastically differently than in our modern world. The physical capability of a 60-year-old hunter-gatherer might be somewhat less than 20 something hunter-gatherers, but the experience and the wisdom will make the elder much more efficient in all aspects of life (including hunting). In a hunter-gatherer's life, aging does not diminish the quality from the years lived as it does in our modern world. There is a relative balance during the entire life when it comes to physical capabilities, and a gradual increase in effectiveness due to more experience and wisdom. In nature there is usually a fast death at the end of life (for example: the leading cause of death amongst hunter-gatherers in Papua New Guinea is to be killed by falling tree branches). In our world people age physically very early and live out an old life for most of their adult lives.

Aging does not need to happen this way, even in modern life, but it requires elevated attention of proper rest and recovery.

Extra note: I came across a common argument, which is that in nature, a long time ago, people lived shorter lives. Looking into the subject in greater depths will make you realize that statistical data on an average life span has little to do with actual individual life span or the success of that lifetime in terms of quality experienced. JFK already realized that "It is not enough for a great nation merely to have added new years to life—our objective must also be to add new life to those years." The death of a newborn added statistically to a long life lived to 100, which statistically averages to only 50. The statistical information doesn't tell the story of the people who grew to adulthood. Our modern emergency medical procedures have improved incredibly, leading to a major drop in child birth death rate, but we grew worse in our own age management.

18. RELATIONSHIP BETWEEN WALKING, RUNNING AND DOING

When an advanced runner comes to me for advice on how to improve their running performance, they often tell me that they run the likes of 50 miles a week, but they feel stuck in a routine, concur injuries from time to time and don't know how to move forward. During my assessment on such runners, I find it interesting that very often they manage to justify running exorbitant distances, but when it comes to walking, they believe it is a waste of time, and practically do not partake whatsoever.

NATURAL ORDER OF MOVEMENT DEVELOPMENT

There is a natural order in capability development as people develop into adults from birth.

First, we learn to do tiny movements as infants, then we learn to crawl, learn to stand, walk and eventually run. Each capability has its base in the previous one and as we want to have a more capable system, we need to be mindful of the natural order.

Yes, you need to be able to walk or hike a fair bit, as well as becoming a good runner. Developing only one aspect of your movement capabilities by pushing your boundaries only in one specific direction, will have a relatively short shelf life in terms of your entire life. Being an active runner for ten years will not contribute much to your overall life, but to be able to do anything for 30, 40, 50 + years you need to use your body with balance in mind.

I am always interested in developing programs for teams and companies where the participants can eventually transfer into an active lifestyle in their personal lives.

Developing and understanding balance for anyone who is interested in a high-quality experience in life will always become very important at one point. You might, for example, reach a stage in your career where doing more will not motivate you anymore, so you might encounter some physical pains, all of which force you to think about your life in terms of what's lacking and what's excessive, so you can find a better balance.

Even professional athletes often times come up against this issue when they retire. Professional athletes' lives are out of balance during their active pro careers, but once the retirement creates the possibility for a better balance, the retired athlete often suffers from finding the 'sweet spot' between staying physically active while allowing other aspects of life to take over the emphasis in their lives. It's the reason so many ex-athletes become fairly out of shape ten years into their retirement – I am sure you can think of a few.

But you don't need to be a pro athlete to have the same issues. You might have an out of balance running regiment because you were part of a running club as a young adult, and once you had kids you could not find the meaning behind activities unless you were pushing yourself to similar levels as when you had nothing else in your life but your running club.

Ask yourself these questions frequently, if you want to have a long-lasting healthy movement regiment: Am I spending too much time n any one type of activity in my life? What is out of balance? Is too much running, or, not running enough; too much exercising, or, too little exercising; too much work, or, too little work; too much socializing, or, too little socializing? Unless you make enough money, you will eventually be worried about not being able to cover your basic needs, which will affect your well-being. If you work too much, eventually you will end up working in ways that start negatively affecting the quality of your life, even if you make more money in the process. Too much socializing cuts into your daily recovery, too little socializing will create a sense of loneliness, which also limits your well-being in the short term, and statistically could be disastrous on the long term.

Identifying too much with one aspect of your life will push you into an out-of-balance state. You are not a runner, you are not an athlete, you are neither a wife, nor a husband, you are not a doctor, nor a taxi driver, nor an artist; these are all only the things you do.

You are first and foremost a human being with multiple different needs. Be grounded and balanced in everything you do.

In a mysterious way, the grounding effect one receives while being connected to the earth with two bare feet, always guides one towards a sense of better balance in their lives. I don't think it is an accident that 'being grounded' is a term used as a description of someone who is stable.

Regardless if you are literal about being 'grounded' or just think about it metaphorically, one thing is certain: the barefoot practitioners I encounter are always people who search for a balanced life.

I believe, if the critical mass of people were practicing in the creation of such balance, the world could be changed from the inside out.

19. CHILD PASSIONS, RELATIONSHIPS & COMMUNAL RUNNING

FEEL LIKE A KID

Most children naturally gravitate towards kicking off their shoes and being barefoot. I grew up in a culture where it was very normal to be barefoot outside between spring and fall, in the rural areas. I remember how I couldn't wait to take my shoes off and feel free at the beginning of the warmer season. The first two weeks of warm weather, while my feet were getting accustomed again to being without shoes after the cold season, were uncomfortable, but every kid knew that each barefoot step got us closer again to enjoying that addictive sense of caressing the ground with our feet – being plugged into nature for a recharge. I loved being barefoot as a youngster. I was lucky enough to find my way back to that joy and was able to lead many people back towards that youthful experience.

It stood out to me how kids always prefer being barefoot, let it be in a gymnastics setting, running around, playing or just scooting around at the beach. The contrast also stands out at how the

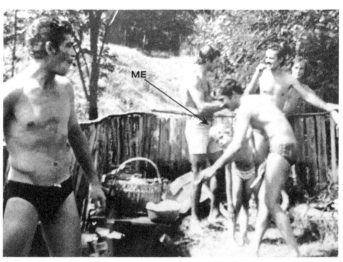

Me with my dad (beside me) and four of my uncles, cooking barefoot, 1979

majority of adults become weirder about being barefoot outside, as they age. Looking at the beautiful foot of a child is an inspiration, seeing the bunion ridden feet of adults is painful. Your adult feet have basically been molded into the shape of a shoe, but it doesn't matter how old you are, you can make a significant difference on how well your foot will age. The choice is yours to let your feet further deteriorate, or you can do things a bit differently and see how you can revitalize them. A stronger, healthier foot has the potential to be the base of a stronger healthier body.

ROLE OF COMMUNAL RUNNING

I urge you not to feel the pressure to become a full-on barefoot exerciser right away, but rather have the goal to dabble into it. Let yourself discover your child-like self again and allow your expectations to naturally change as you gain more understanding and experience in being barefoot.

I ask involved runners regularly about the significant amount of alone time they spend away from home while on runs. The answers are always similar: "My wife doesn't like it" or, "My boyfriend is annoyed by it."

Inspire others who you believe could also become interested in joining on this new journey into well-being. I run a lot - some might even say an extreme amount. I also exercise and do other sports. But there is nothing I enjoy more than when I run with my wife, my kids, my parents, my in-laws, my sister, nieces, nephew, my brother-in-law, my co-workers or my friends. I've only managed to do this communal running irregularly due to having our family life split between North America and Europe, but when we manage to organize it, it feels like the complete wellness experience. It took me and my family time to build an active tribe, but it was well worth it. I urge you to do your best to involve more of your loved ones in your wellness journey.

I believe that running has had a huge role in the development of my exceptional relationship with wife. We probably run together more often than other couples even see each other. We talk and we practice silence, we argue and we resolve, we theorize and we laugh;

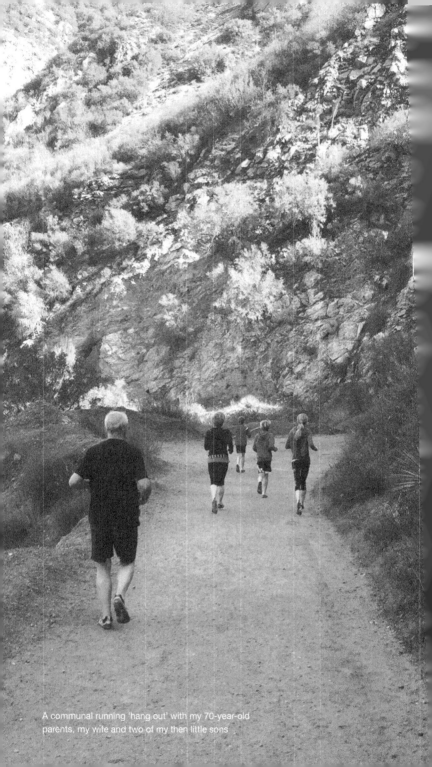

A communal running 'hang out' with my 70-year-old parents, my wife and two of my then little sons nd all this while we run. I bet most couples therapy sessions, and ivorces, could be avoided if couples would spend more active time ogether, especially in nature. It is no accident that bonding chemicals oxytocin, etc.) release while we do cardiovascular activities, because ve were wired to bond together with whom we sweat together - our very own Persistence Hunter Tribe. Bond with physical activities, to hose with whom you want to have a good relationship.

t is no accident that people can maintain a steady, long distance ohysical capability in running, throughout most of their lives. According to related studies in natural environments, young adults in their late teens and the elderly in their 60s have very similar endurance capabilities. It is a tool that exists for us to use not only for hunting, but perhaps also to create well-functioning families, which could lead to a better overall society.

There is a high probability, that during our evolutionary past as hunter-gatherer families, tribes ran together as part of their persistence hunting process to hunt more effectively. Everyone was participating for different reasons. The elders were able to bring their wisdom of tracking and taught the younger ones during the hunt. The most physically capable adults, the middle-aged ones, were able to pursue the chase when there was the need to scare the animal, by sprinting at them – so the animal didn't have the chance to stop for long enough to recover. And at the end of the hunt, when the tribe succeeded, they all ate together, joyously feasting on a kudu or an eland, for example.

You can also try to mimic this experience by running in communities with people you care about. People enjoy running events even when they aren't familiar with most of the participants. Imagine how it would feel to have partners in barefoot runs with some of the people you care about. You can even make it a tradition to finish a nice long run with a group lunch, mimicking the old ways of hunting.

Do not participate only in barefoot activities for the sake of your individual health, but lead by example with those activities for your loved ones. When you do so, others will join you and it will provide extra meaning in your physically active lifestyle.

20. IN CLOSING

I was always fascinated by science. When I was younger, I looked towards science to guide me and give me ideas about what to experiment with and how. As I've grown older, wiser and more experienced, my relationship with science has changed.

Today I keep up with science mostly because I am curious to see if science will catch up to what I've seen working well throughout the years to enhance the human experience. I used to feel strange announcing this very notion to others until I realized that most health practitioners with longevity shared the same views.

When it comes to barefoot running, its benefits and full importance are still missing - mostly in scientific circles. The reason for this is perhaps because being barefoot cannot be just a theory. Being barefoot must be practiced and experienced to feel it, subconsciously at first in the body, and only then gradually develop an awareness of its components and benefits consciously, as well. There are some interesting and encouraging studies that have emerged during the past decades from the University of Harvard in regards to barefoot existence - and even on persistence hunting. I hope that this handbook will trigger your interest as a newly practicing barefoot runner; and also bring out in you, the theorizing scientist as well.

The more of us who return to practicing human activities the way we were designed to practice, the more of us will connect directly to Earth. Perhaps when we connect with our bare feet to Mother Earth, we can all show our appreciation and care towards her more.

In the near future our care towards Earth may become an absolute necessity for our very existence, and not just a philosophical discussion.

A barefoot that is grounded in nature always carries a head high up that is interested in conserving nature. The separation between the body's inner environment and the body's outer environment blurs more and more with each barefoot step, and eventually leads us to the necessary understanding that without direct connection to Nature, there will eventually be no people.

Let your bare feet take you not only towards your healthier future, but towards a healthier future for all living things.

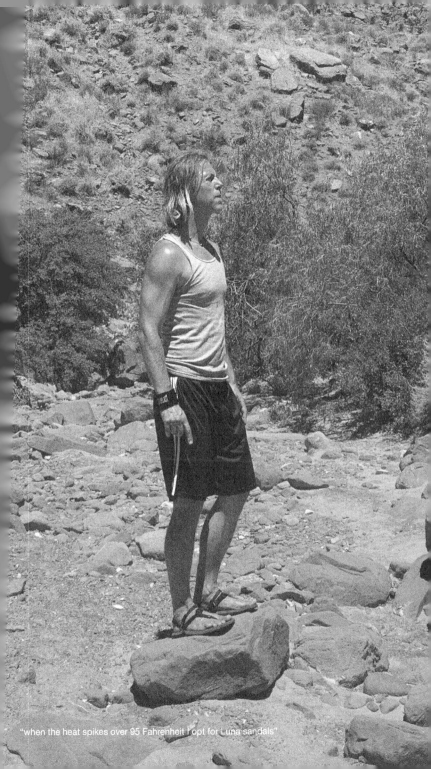

"when the heat spikes over 95 Fahrenheit I opt for Luna sandals"

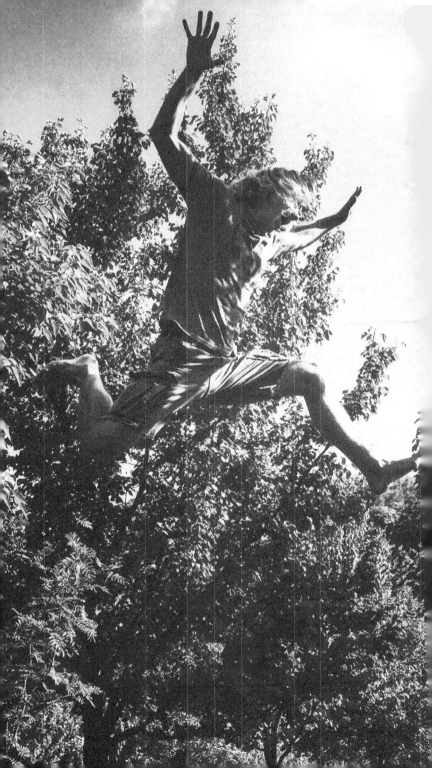

I. PROGRESSIVE BAREFOOT DEVELOPMENT

PROGRAM OUTLINE

This is a general guideline based on my experience of how an interested individual without any major biomechanical injuries, could start running barefoot from scratch. One might ask what is the difference between an experienced runner's process versus a complete beginner. The structure of the process must be very similar. In my experience, the only difference is that an experienced runner will be able to go through each individual step of the outline exactly as described, while a novice runner might need to randomly repeat many of the individual steps.

PHASE I.

(WALKING)

Start out by walking barefoot first, to build barefoot capability.

Start with 10 minutes of barefoot walking. As long as you do not experience any joint or foot pain, during or after the walk, add 2 minutes to the length of your next barefoot walk. Keep increasing the amount of time you spend walking barefoot by 2 minutes, as long as you have no discomfort.

In the case you experience some discomfort, don't increase your walking time until you can manage to do the same length of barefoot walking without any discomfort. Only then increase the amount of time you spend on walking barefoot, by two minutes.

You can walk daily. Vary the surface you walk upon – do not get stuck on the exact same surface for every walk.

Work up your capability of pain-free barefoot walking to at least one hour.

Once you have reached this first cornerstone, you can try implementing some running into your regiment.

PHASE II.

(WALK/RUN)

For the first session, gently test the capability of your foot and follow the structure of 1 minute walking then switch into 1 minute 'easy run'. I would warn against doing more than 6 segments of this walking/running (12 minute) cycle the first time around. Being conservative is wise, because rushing things will only expose you to a higher chance of pain and discomfort. At the end of each running session, you want to finish on a high note so that you feel excited about the next run. Grow your capabilities, slowly – within a month or so you will grow your process to a more impressive level, even this way.

If you have **no muscle ache** or muscle soreness the next day, after the first barefoot running work out, then add an additional two segments the next time you do the work out. Continue adding 2 segments (4 minutes) to your barefoot walk/run process, every time. Again, the emphasis is that there must not be any muscle nor joint aches, or any other discomforts present. If you experience any muscle or joint aches, during or after your work out, then the next time just stick with the same number of segments you did previously, without pain. Eventually you will be able to push out that threshold and complete the extra segments without any discomfort. Only run at a pace that you can still manage to breathe exclusively through your nose. This will be a good guide for your entire start-out process.

Leave 48 hours for your body to recover in between two of these barefoot walking/running sessions.

Once you have worked up to 15 segments (30 minutes) of the 1-minute walking and 1-minute running you can move into the next phase.

PHASE III.

(RUNNING EXTENSIONS WITH WALKING RECOVERY)

During this phase you want to increase the amount of barefoot running you do, while still breaking up the running segments with walking 'resting-periods'.

First, do 2 minutes of running followed by 1 minute walking (3-minute segment) and repeat this 10 times (making it into a 30-minute barefoot activity).

If you experience even the slightest foot, Achilles-tendon, shin muscle soreness or any joint aches do NOT add more cycles to your program until you can manage the same segment without any discomfort.

Once you have gone through all the three phases, continue the progression with the following process, as noted in the chart below:

	Walking Time (minutes)	Running Time (minutes)	Segments	Workout Time (minutes
Session 1	1	2	10	30
Session 2	1	3	7	28
Session 3	1	4	6	30
Session 4	1	5	5	30
Session 5	1	6	4	28
Session 6	1	7	4	32
Session 7	1	8	3	27
Session 8	1	9	3	30
Session 9	1	10	3	33
Session 10	1	15	2	32

Finish this phase with a non-stop 30 minute barefoot run and move onto the next phase.

PHASE IV.

(RUNNING)

During this phase the goal is to increase the amount of time you spend barefoot running.

You should now have the capability to run barefoot for 30 minutes with no problem. Increase the length of your run by 5 minutes each time until you make it up to 90 minutes.

This might sound very easy, but certain segments of this process might drag out longer than you would expect. The reason for this might be physical, but it could also be how much time you are able to devote to your running regiment out of your schedule.

At this stage, running 3-4 times a week is good. You want to make sure you run at least 2 times per week otherwise you will not provide enough stimuli to your body to respond to improvement.

PHASE V.

(PERSISTENCE RUNNING)

Based on all the research and experience, which I have gathered, human being should have the capability to run at least a 1.5 Marathon distance (approximately 40 miles or so). There is limited actual data available on persistence hunting, however based on years of analysis of the available scientific information (listening to countless stories of hunter-gatherer anecdotes and my first-hand experience in practicing and coaching persistence running) allows me to speculate that human beings (homo sapiens sapiens, homo sapiens neanderthalensis and all the other mysterious other homo sapiens that once existed) are designed to be able to run down most animals in elevated heat to the point of exhaustion as long as the hunter can manage to keep up after them for up to about 40 miles.

Once someone has achieved this barefoot running capability in our modern world, I don't believe it should be continuously practiced all year long. Instead, set out to focus on it for about 3-4 months out of the year. The remaining seasons of the year should be spent with many other physically active, but not running focused, sporting activities. Persistence hunting was a seasonal hunting method, which gave our ancestors enough time to recover from the elevated running demands between each persistence running season.

It takes a while to work up to the running capability of performing such long-distance barefoot activities (even most runners with shoes never experience running this long).

This progress outline is far from a complete program that is the perfect fit for everyone. My goal with the outline is to make sure that the method of structuring the program is communicated. Working with an experienced coach is always a wise way to customize your individual running process.

II. RUNNER'S BASIC SUPPORTING EXERCISES

You are also able to find a video explanation of all the followings exercises on www.coachbarefoot.com/book.

INCH WORM

It is difficult to consciously learn a movement, which is naturally learned prior to developing any capability of conscious activities. This is such an ancient type of movement that we are instinctually wired to start practicing it very early on, at the beginning of the newborn phase of our lives.

POSITIONING:

Lay down on a hard, smooth surface. A carpet or a yoga mat will be fine.

Cross your arms over your chest. Make sure you do NOT use your shoulders in any form for this exercise. In the beginning the temptation to roll onto the shoulders will be huge, for most people.

Lift up your legs and bend your knees.

This exercise has two different phases to it.

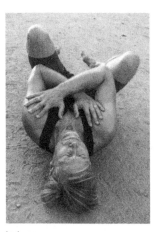

Inch worm

Phase I: moving towards the direction of the head

Imagine that you have a downward-pointing hook attached to the back of your head.

Dig that hook into the ground and pull yourself along the ground with the help of your head.

Each time when you pull with the back of your head using your neck, simultaneously you have to pull

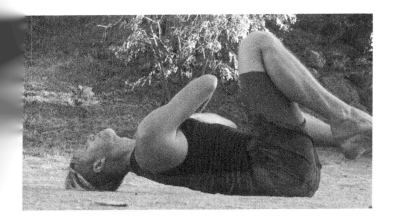

your back up into an arch and also move one of your hips upwards by tilting yourself a little sideways (remember not to roll on to your shoulder).

Then, you want to readjust your neck with the imaginary hook and reach further up, arching up the spine again and lift the other hip up, inching it closer to the direction of the head.

Continue moving in this sequence, inching yourself upwards, over the ground as an inch worm would do it.

Phase II: moving towards the direction of the legs

On the way down you do not need to do the side angulation and you are only moving your body in a straight line.

Shorten the back of your neck by lifting up your chin – but keep your head on the ground.

Shift weight onto the back of your head and lift up your entire back into an arch, only the back of your head and the back of your pelvis are touching the ground.

Now tuck your chin in and at the same time, tilt your pelvis backwards and push your entire body along the floor for a few inches.

The next movement starts again by shortening the neck, lifting the chin and tilting your pelvis forward.

You are moving like an inch worm along the floor.

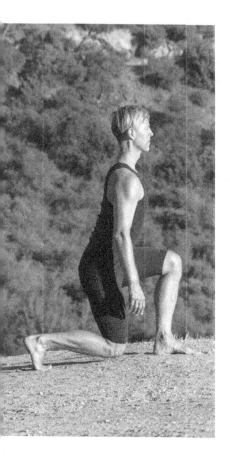
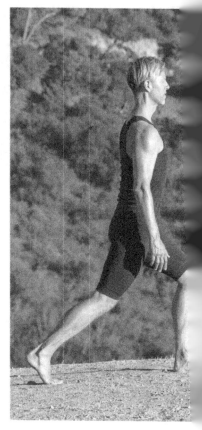

LUNGES

Both feet need to point forward perfectly – do not let the back foot point outwards.

Make sure you have a bit more weight on the heel of the front foot.

Imagine you are moving up and down along a plumber's line – do not shift your body weight back and forth.

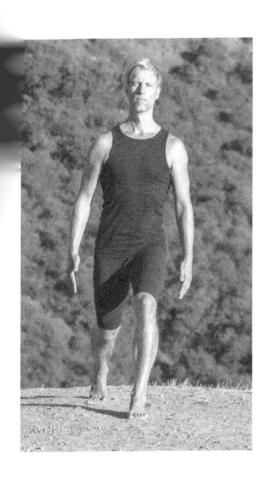

Look straight ahead.

Do not let your front knee move further forward than your toes.

Keep the second toe of your front foot, the middle of the knee of the front leg and the center of the front hip aligned.

MAASAI JUMPING

Keep jumping up and down in the same spot.

Keep looking straight ahead, so your body is always taking off in a straight upward trajectory.

Most of the movement is coming from your feet, ankles and your knees.

You can try using your spine as part of the spring mechanism that generates the force in between jumps.

It is a continuous, non-stop movement.

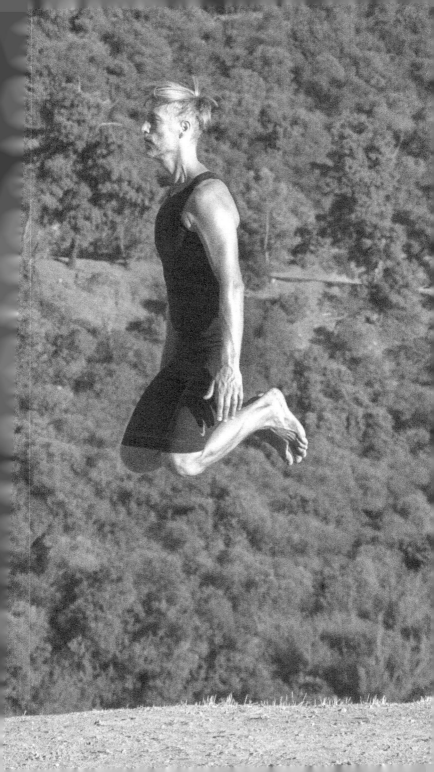

SOVIET LADDER

Climb up on the first step of the ladder, facing away from the ladder.

Jump off the ladder onto a hard surface.

Only increase the height of the step you are using to jump off, if you have completed a full work out session and experienced no pain whatsoever during, nor after the exercise session.

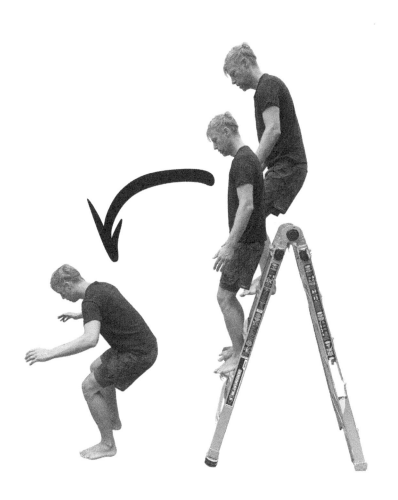

III. RUNNER'S BASIC STRETCHES

There are also video explanations of the following stretches on www.coachbarefoot.com/book.

These stretches are not by any means a complete list of stretches a runner should practice, but many of the stretches must be individualized based on your body's personal history. The following list contains stretching movements, which I find very useful, in general, for many people.

In the case you have any history of disc degeneration or discomfort resulting in altering your way of movement, I would highly recommend to find a good health practitioner to support, guide and structure your individualized procedures to achieve your physical health goals.

Correct body positioning is key with any stretching. Always start nice and gently with any exercise and slowly experiment with them to see how they affect your body.

VERTICAL L STRETCH

A fascia stretching movement will feel like a hard isometric exercise instead of a usual stretch, at least until you get good at it. This exercise might not only improve your mobility, but will also strengthen some of the necessary postural muscles in your body to have a more stable structure.

This is only one of many of these types of stretches, which a person could benefit from using. In the case you are interested in effective fascia stretches I would recommend looking into learning ELDOA stretches from a practitioner.

Once you have placed yourself into the position of this stretch, I recommend you work up the capability to hold this position for 1 minute. Make sure you do not hold your breath while performing any stretching movements.

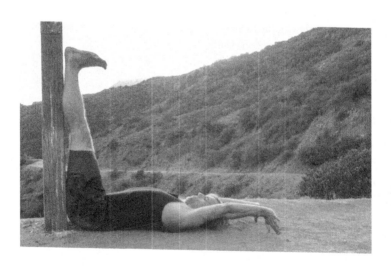

ay down on your back and get your buttocks as close as possible
o a tree or a wall.

Put your legs up on the wall, so your legs are basically perpendicular
o the floor.

Ideally you want to have your legs so straight on the wall that your
heels are not touching the wall. For most people this is a high order
o start with, but try and work yourself up to that capability, over
time.

Lift up your arms straight over your head and keep them as close to
the ground as possible.

Rotate your arms outward as much as possible and open your
hands and spread your fingers as wide as possible, while extending
your wrist into a 90-degree position.

At the same time, dorsi-flex your ankle so your feet are facing up to
the ceiling.

Keep this up throughout the entire stretch.

Flatten your lower back to the ground.

You want to try relaxing your abdominals as much as possible.

Tuck your chin, keep your head on the ground.

Push your head away from the body maintaining the above
position.

As you try this stretching exercise you will notice that your entire
body feels like it has tensed up, but make sure to keep elevated
attention on keeping your quadriceps and the front part of your
shin area, contracted. Keep trying to push your upper limbs away
from the wall and simultaneously keep pushing the legs away from
the ground towards the ceiling.

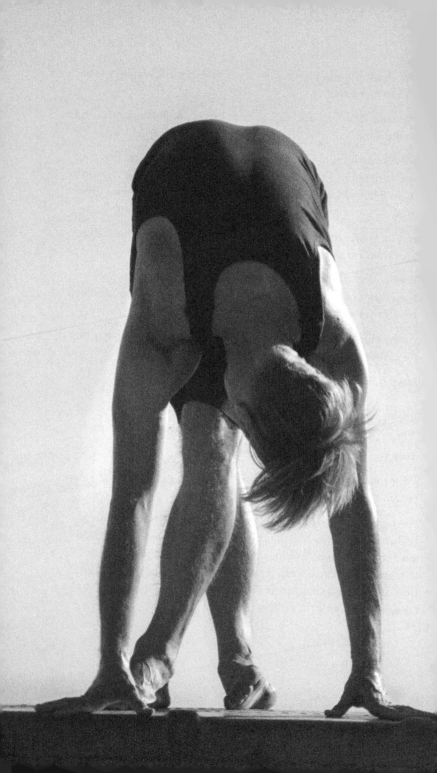

STANDING SWAN STRETCH

Start the stretch standing upright.

Put one leg behind the other, crossing the legs, and at the same time put the back ankle into a 'twisted' position (just like when someone 'twists' their ankle). At this point the 'twisted' foot is going to be facing away from the body, the outside of the ankle facing down to the ground.

Turn your upper body towards the same direction your 'twisted' foot is facing.

Then, start bending down and reach with your arms towards the ground.

With each exhalation attempt to gently get closer to the ground.

Eventually you might be able to even place your palms on the ground while stretching.

Hold this stretch for a minimum of 8-16 full breaths, then repeat the same thing on the other side.

STANDING NUMBER 4 STRETCH

From an upright standing position, lift up one leg and place the outside of the ankle on the other thigh, right above the knee (you will look as if you were the number 4).

You can hold onto the lower part of the bent leg.

Push your buttocks back as if you are trying to sit back down while maintaining your normal lower back position (do not let your spine flex forward much).

Keep the back of your neck long.

Hold this stretch for a minimum of 8-16 full breaths, then repeat the same thing on the other side.

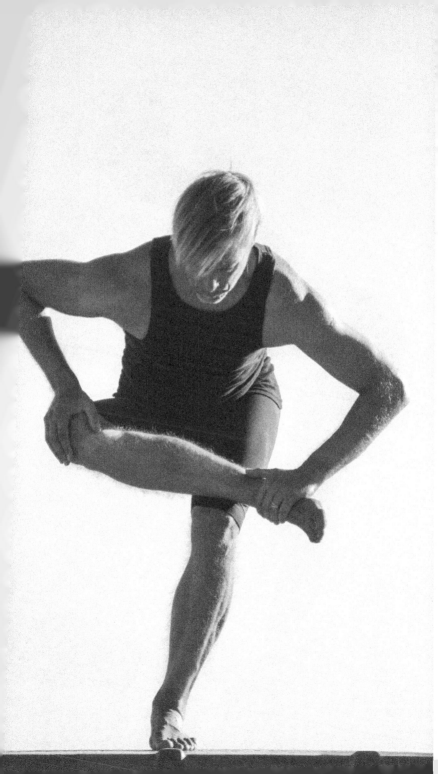

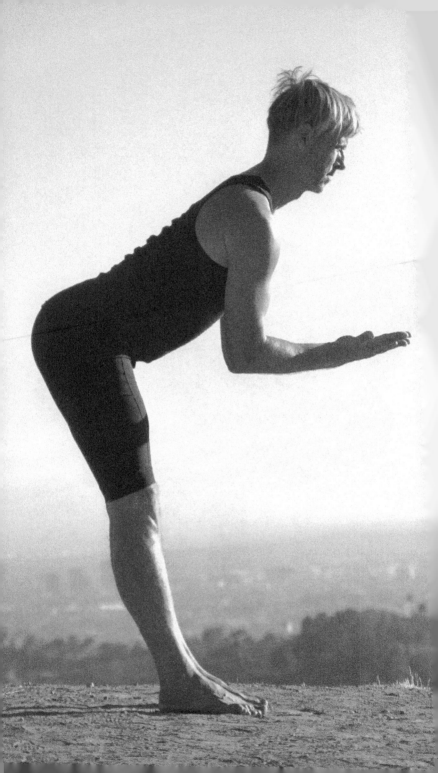

SERVANT'S BOW STRETCH

From an upright standing position, imagine you were a servant in front of a king.

Make sure your feet are hip width distance, symmetric, and pointing forward.

Keep your lower back slightly arched and tilt your torso forward from the hips.

Go as deep as you can manage without altering the arch in your lower back.

You can pinch the skin on your lower back to make sure you don't lose your lower back position.

ENGLISH SPLIT STAND STRETCH

Step into a long split stand position.

Keep the front foot flat on the ground, while pushing down the heel of the back foot as close to the ground as possible.

Place your hands flat on the ground beside each other on the inside of the front leg.

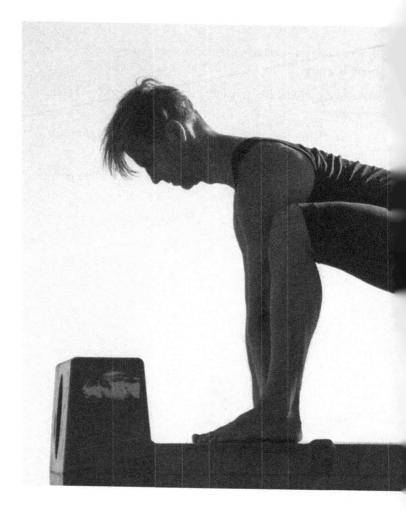

Keep the back of the neck long and keep your back straight.

Hold this stretch for a minimum of 8-16 full breaths, then repeat the same thing on the other side.

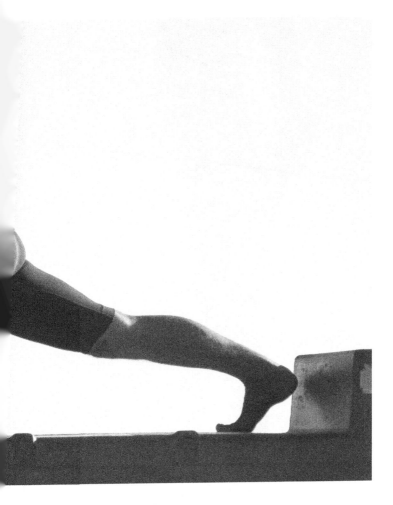

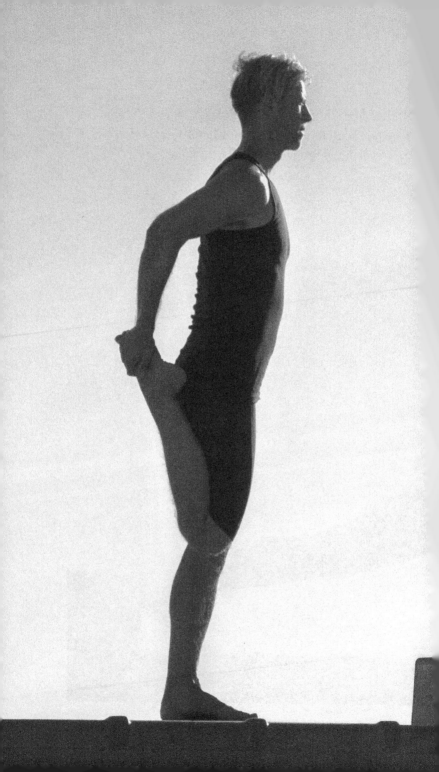

FLAMINGO STRETCH

From an upright standing position, pick up one leg, bend the knee and grab the ankle of that leg, pulling it towards your buttocks.

Keep your knees beside each other.

Pull the heel of the bent leg as close to your buttocks as possible.

Keep looking straight ahead.

Contract your buttock muscles on the side of the bent leg.

Hold this stretch for a minimum of 8-16 full breaths, then repeat the same thing on the other side.

PUSHING THE WALL STRETCH

Place your hands on a solid vertical object (a tree or a wall).

Step back with one straight leg, but only as far as you can still manage (barely) to flatten the back foot to the ground.

Make sure both feet are pointing perfectly forward.

Try continuously straightening the back knee and pushing the heel of the back foot into the ground.

Hold this stretch for a minimum of 8-16 full breaths, then repeat the same thing on the other side.

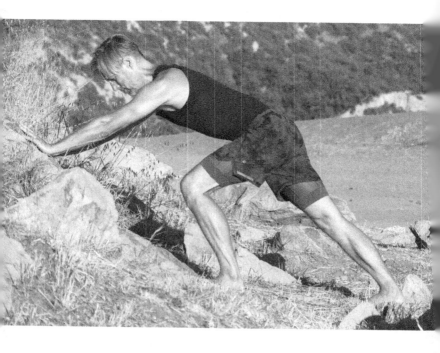

DEEP SQUAT STRETCH

Hang onto a solid object (a tree for example).

Step a little wider than your hips.

Make sure your feet are symmetric – they should NOT be parallel (feet should slightly point outward)!

Squat down as deep as you can while holding onto the solid object.

Make sure to keep your feet flat on the ground.

Your 2nd toe, the middle of your knee caps and your hips should be aligned on both sides.

Go only as deep as you can manage while still maintaining proper alignment (outlined above).

Hold your deepest squatting position for a minimum of 8-16 full breaths.

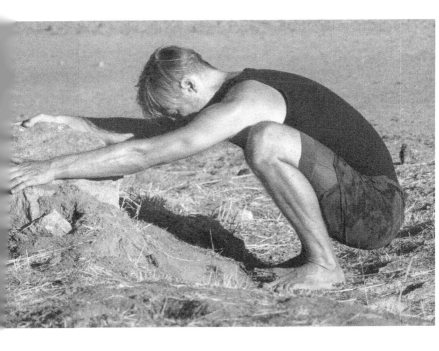

CSABA'S RECOMMENDED
BOOK REFERENCE GUIDE

Affluence without Abundance by James Suzman

Barefoot Running: Step by Step by Barefoot Ken Bob Saxton

Born To Run by Christopher McDougall

Epic Survival by Matt Graham

Finding Ultra by Rich Roll

How to Eat, Move and Be Healthy by Paul Chek

Manthropology by Peter McAllister

Mechanical Low Back Pain by James Porterfield

Supertraining by Yuri V. Verkhoshansky, Mel C. Siff

The Art of Tracking by Louis Liebenberg

Les ELDOA by Guy Voyer

The Story of the Human Body by Daniel E. Lieberman

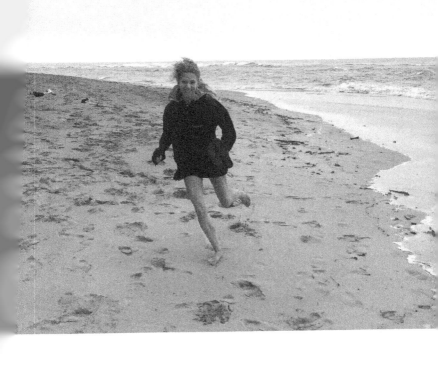

IV. ACKNOWLEDGEMENTS

Many thanks to all those whose work, experience, research and support helped me to write and complete this book, especially Winter Ave Zoli, Marney Stratton, Susann Lucas, Gina Star, Christina Ulloa, Andrea Szőcs, Chris Maund and the remote Bushman of Botswana and Namibia.

I would also like to thank my kids, Tristan, Atreyu, Wilder and Anick, who were my ultimate motivators to write down my experiences.

And finally, but not least, I am happy to have the opportunity to thank my parents, Ella & Csaba Szőcs, who have always been my biggest supporters in anything I set out to do - including to speak and write in English.

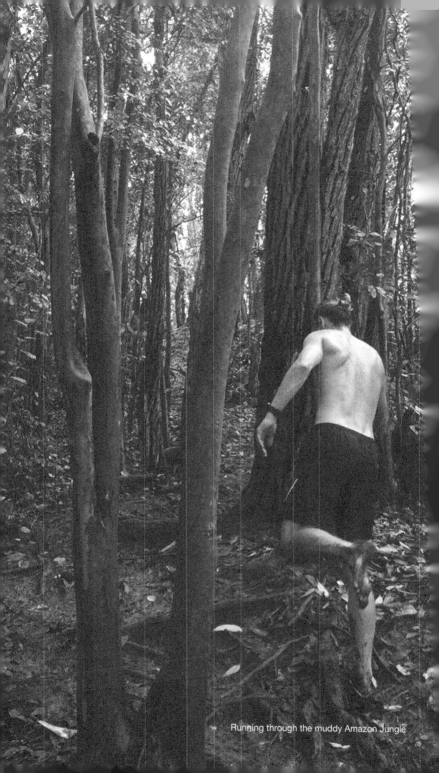
Running through the muddy Amazon Jungle

DISCLAIMER

Although the publisher and the author have made every effort to ensure that the information in this book was correct at press time and while this publication is designed to provide accurate information in regard to the subject matter covered, the publisher and the author assume no responsibility for errors, inaccuracies, omissions, or any other inconsistencies herein and hereby disclaim any liability to any party for any loss, damage, or disruption caused by errors or omissions, whether such errors or omissions result from negligence, accident, or any other cause.

The publisher and the author make no guarantees concerning the level of success you may experience by following the advice and strategies contained in this book, and you accept the risk that results will differ for each individual. The testimonials and examples provided in this book show exceptional results, which may not apply to the average reader, and are not intended to represent or guarantee that you will achieve the same or similar results. All information contained in this book publication is provided "as is" and the publisher and the author make no representations or warranties of any kind with respect of the book's contents.

The author of this book is not a professional and the content of this book publication is being provided for informational purposes only.

The information contained in this book publication is no substitute for direct expert assistance and, if such assistance is required, the services of a competent professional should be sought.

Any references to other published work in this book publication was provided for convenience only and the publisher and the author make no warranties or representation as to the accuracy of that information.

The statements made about products and services have not been evaluated by the U.S. Food and Drug Administration. They are not intended to diagnose, treat, cure, or prevent any condition or disease. Please consult with your own physician or healthcare specialist regarding the suggestions and recommendations made in this book.

Except as specifically stated in this book, neither the author or publisher, nor any authors, contributors, or other representatives will be liable for damages arising out of or in connection with the use of this book.

This is a comprehensive limitation of liability that applies to all damages of any kind, including (without limitation) compensatory; direct, indirect or consequential damages; loss of data, income or profit; loss of or damage to property and claims of third parties.

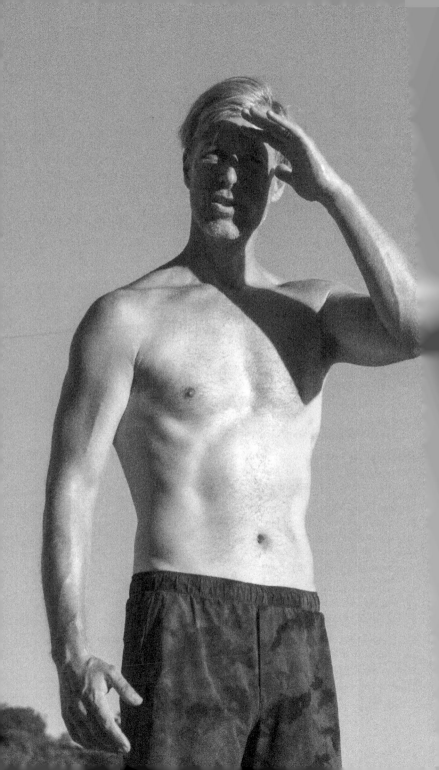

ABOUT THE AUTHOR

'Coach Barefoot', Csaba Lucas, is a Hungarian author, coach, speaker, extreme adventure guide and business advisor. Csaba resides in Los Angeles, California and has been a health coach for the past 30 years. Csaba lives as a 21st century Renaissance man, applying his unique approach of bringing the ancient traditions of the past into our modern-day present lives. Csaba oversees the services of his coaching company (Modern Age Warriors). These services range from bringing resolutions to corporate business conflicts, leading clients on extreme adventure trips, and consulting with his clients to aid them in bringing success, happiness, health and fulfillment to every aspect of their lives. Csaba is happily married and is the proud father of four.

connect with me
@coachbarefoot.com

Made in the USA
Las Vegas, NV
28 August 2022

54234767R00070